Alternative Medicine: Beginners Guide to Alternative Medicine

A wide-ranging guide to a number of the disparate techniques that come under the umbrella of alternative and complementary medicine. Over twenty therapies and techniques are clearly explained, including the Alexander technique, chiropractic, homeopathy, colour therapy, naturopathy, dance movement therapy, auricular therapy, and many more.

Contents

An Introduction to Alternative Medicine

'Alternative medicine' is a commonly used general term to describe ·all the methods of healing other than those practised by conventional doctors working in general practice or in hospitals. Most people become very familiar with the methods of conventional or orthodox medicine but are less informed about alternative therapies. This may be due partly to the fact that a bewildering variety of alternative therapies exists. However, a more significant factor is almost certainly that, until very recently, methods of alternative medicine were regarded with complete scepticism by much of the medical and scientific establishment. Attitudes have gradually become more enlightened (although doubts still exist in some quarters), and there has been a growing realization that alternative therapies have much to offer in the common aim of helping and healing patients.

Many forms of alternative medicine exist, some being complete methods in themselves, involving both diagnosis and treatment, while others are complementary to conventional practice. An example of the former is homoeopathy while massage and aromatherapy fall into the latter category. Some methods of alternative therapy require a period of training at a recognized establishment, which may last for some years and is often undertaken by those with existing medical or nursing qualifications. For other methods, a relatively short training course is needed and the practitioner is not expected to possess medical knowledge to any great extent.

Some alternative therapies have been practised for centuries and date back to the earliest known human civilizations. This is hardly surprising when it is considered that it is orthodox medicine that is, in fact, relatively new, especially in the form in which it is known today. That which is now regarded as "alternative" may have been the only form of treatment available to people in the past.

In this book, the most well-known and widely practised forms of alternative medicine are described in some detail and other methods are also mentioned. The book does not claim to cover the subject in full detail and some methods have been omitted. It is recommended that a person seeking alternative therapy in any form should obtain advice and as much information as possible, and first consult their own general practitioner.

Acupressure

This is an ancient form of healing combining massage and acupuncture, practised over 3,000 years ago in Japan and China. It was developed into its current form using a system of special massage points and is today still practised widely in the Japanese home environment.

Certain 'pressure points' are located in various parts of the body and these are used by the practitioner by massaging firmly with the thumb or fingertip. These points are the same as those utilized in acupuncture. There are various ways of working and the pressure can be applied by the practitioner's fingers, thumbs, knees, palms of the hand, etc. Relief from pain can be quite rapid at times, depending upon its cause, while other more persistent problems can take longer to improve.

Acupressure is said to enhance the body's own method of healing, thereby preventing illness and improving the energy level. The pressure exerted is believed to regulate a matter called 'Qi', which is energy that flows along 'meridians'. These are invisible channels that run along the length of the body. These meridians are mainly named after the organs of the body such as the liver and stomach, but there are four exceptions, which are called the 'pericardium" 'triple heater', 'conception' and 'governor'. Specifically named meridian lines may also be used to treat ailments other than those relating to it.

Ailments claimed to have been treated successfully are back pain, asthma, digestive problems, insomnia, migraine and circulatory problems, amongst others. Changes in diet, regular exercise and certain self-checking methods may be recommended by your practitioner. It must be borne in mind that some painful symptoms are the onset of serious illness so you should always first consult your Doctor.

Before any treatment commences, a patient will be asked details of lifestyle and diet, the pulse rate will be taken along with any relevant past history relating to the current problem. The person will be requested to lie on a mattress on the floor or on a firm table, and comfortable but loose-fitting clothing is best so that the practitioner can work most effectively on the energy channels. No oils are used on the body and there is no equipment. Each session lasts from approximately 30 minutes to I hour. Once the pressure is applied, and this can be done in a variety of ways particular to each practitioner, varying sensations may be felt. Some points may feel sore or tender and there may be some discomfort such as a deep pain or coolness. However, it is believed that this form of massage works quickly so that any tenderness soon passes.

The number of treatments will vary from patient to patient, according to how the person responds and what problem or ailment is being treated. Weekly visits may be needed if a specific disorder is being treated while other people may go whenever they feel in need. It is advisable for women who are pregnant to check with their practitioner first since some of the acupressure methods are not recommended during pregnancy. Acupressure can be practised safely at home although it is usually better for one person to perform the massage on another. Common problems such as headache, constipation and toothache can be treated quite simply although there is the possibility of any problem worsening first before an improvement occurs if the pressure points are over stimulated. You should, however, see your doctor if any ailment persists. To treat headache, facial soreness, toothache and menstrual pain, locate the fleshy piece of skin between the thumb and forefinger and squeeze firmly, pressing towards the forefinger. The pressure should be applied for about five minutes and either hand can be used. This point is known as 'Large Intestine 4'.

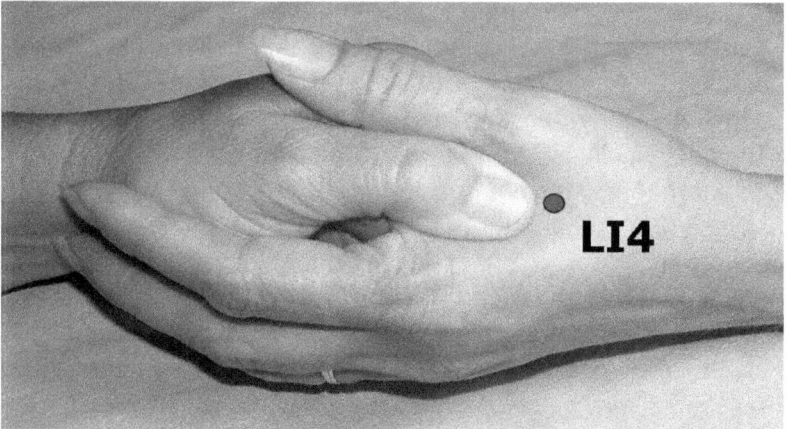

Large Intestine 4

To aid digestive problems in both adults and babies, for example to settle infantile colic, the point known as 'Stomach 36' is utilized, which is located on the outer side of the leg about 75mm (3ins) down from the knee. This point should be quite simple to find as it can often feel slightly tender. It should be pressed quite firmly and strongly for about five to ten minutes with the thumb.

When practising acupressure massage on someone else and before treatment begins, ensure that the person is warm, relaxed, comfortable and wearing loose-fitting clothing and that he or she is lying on a firm mattress or rug on the floor. To discover the areas that need to be worked on, press firmly over the body and see which areas are tender. These tender areas on the body correspond to an organ that is not working correctly. To commence massage using fingertips or thumbs, a pressure of about 4.5 kg (10 lbs) should be exerted. The massage movements should be performed very quickly, about 50 to 100 times every minute, and some discomfort is likely (which will soon pass) but there should be no pain. Particular care should be taken to avoid causing pain on the face, stomach or over any joints. If a baby or young child is being massaged then considerably less pressure should be used. If there is any doubt as to the correct amount, exert a downwards pressure on bathroom scales to ascertain the weight being used.

There is no need to hurry from one point to another since approximately 5 to 15 minutes is needed at each point for adults, but only about 30 seconds for babies or young children.

Using the 'self-help' acupressure, massage can be repeated as often as is felt to be necessary with several sessions per hour usually being sufficient for painful conditions that have arisen suddenly. It is possible that as many as 20 sessions may be necessary for persistent conditions causing pain, with greater intervals of time between treatments as matters improve. It is not advisable to try anything that is at all complicated (or to treat an illness such as arthritis) and a trained practitioner will obviously be able to provide the best level of treatment and help. To contact a reputable practitioner who has completed the relevant training it is advisable to contact the appropriate professional body.

Acupuncture

This is an ancient Chinese therapy that involves inserting needles into the skin at specific points of the body. The word 'acupuncture' originated from a Dutch physician, William Ten

Rhyne, who had been living in Japan during the latter part of the 17th century and it was he who introduced it to Europe. The term means literally 'prick with a needle'. The earliest textbook on acupuncture, dating from approximately 400 BC, was called *Nei Ching Su Wen,* which means 'Yellow Emperor's Classic of Internal Medicine'.

Also recorded at about the same time was the successful saving of a patient's life by acupuncture, the person having been expected to die whilst in a coma. Legend has it that acupuncture was developed when it was realized that soldiers who recovered from arrow wounds were sometimes also healed of other diseases from which they were suffering. Acupuncture was very popular with British doctors in the early 1800s for pain relief and to treat fever. There was also a specific article on the successful treatment of rheumatism that appeared in *The Lancet.* Until the end of the Ching dynasty in China in 1911, acupuncture was slowly developed and improved, but then medicine from the West increased in popularity.

However, more recently there has been a revival of interest and it is again widely practised throughout China. Also, nowadays the use of laser beams and electrical currents are found to give an increased stimulative effect when using acupuncture needles.

The specific points of the body into which acupuncture needles are inserted are located along 'meridians'. These are the pathways or energy channels and are believed to be related to the internal organs of the body. This energy is known as *qi* and the needles are used to decrease or increase the flow of energy, or to unblock it if it is impeded. Traditional Chinese medicine sees the body as being comprised of two natural forces known as the *yin* and *yang*. These two forces are complementary to each other but also opposing, the yin being the female force and calm and passive and also representing the dark, cold, swelling and moisture. The yang force is the male and is stimulating and aggressive, representing the heat and light, contraction and dryness.

It is believed that the cause of ailments and diseases is due to an imbalance of these forces in the body, e.g. if a person is suffering from a headache or high blood pressure then this is because of an excess of yang. If, however, there is an excess of yin, this might result in tiredness, feeling cold and fluid retention.

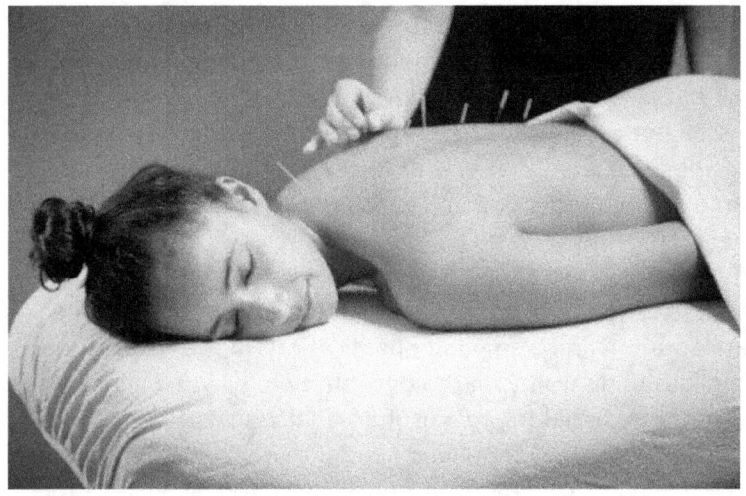

The aim of acupuncture is to establish that there is an imbalance of yin and yang and to rectify it by using the needles at certain points on the body. Traditionally there were 365 points but more have been found in the intervening period and nowadays there can be as many as 2,000. There are 14 meridians, called after the organs they represent, e.g. the lung, kidney, heart and stomach as well as two organs unknown in orthodox medicine-the triple heater or warmer, which relates to the activity of the endocrine glands and the control of temperature. In addition, the pericardium is concerned with seasonal activity and also regulates the circulation of the blood. Of the 14 meridians, there are two, known as the *du,* or governor, and the *ren,* or conception, which both run straight up the body's midline, although the du is much shorter, extending from the head down to the mouth, while the ren starts at the chin and extends to the base of the trunk.

There are several factors that can change the flow of qi (also known as shi orch'i), and they can be of an emotional, physical or environmental nature. The flow may be changed to become too slow or fast, or it can be diverted or blocked so that the incorrect organ is involved and the acupuncturist has to ensure that the flow returns to normal. There are many painful afflictions for which acupuncture can be used. In the West, it has been used primarily for rheumatism, back pain and arthritis, but it has also been used to alleviate other disorders such as stress, allergy, colitis, digestive troubles, insomnia, asthma, etc. It has been claimed that withdrawal symptoms (experienced by people stopping smoking and ceasing other forms of addiction) have been helped as well.

Qualified acupuncturists complete a training course of three years duration and also need qualifications in the related disciplines of anatomy, pathology, physiology and diagnosis before they can belong to a professional association. It is very important that a fully qualified acupuncturist, who is a member of the relevant professional body, is consulted because at the present time, any unqualified person can use the title 'acupuncturist'.

At a consultation, the traditional acupuncturist uses a set method of ancient rules to determine the acupuncture points. The texture and colouring of the skin, type of skin, posture and movement and the tongue will all be examined and noted, as will the patient's voice. These different factors are all needed for the Chinese diagnosis. A number of questions will be asked concerning the diet, amount of exercise taken, lifestyle, fears and phobias, sleeping patterns and reactions to stress. Each wrist has six pulses, and each of these stand for a main organ and its function. The pulses are felt (known as palpating), and by this means acupuncturists are able to diagnose any problems relating to the flow of qi and if there is any disease present in the internal organs. The needles used in acupuncture are disposable and made of a fine stainless steel and come already sealed in a sterile pack. They can be sterilized by the acupuncturist in a machine known as an autoclave but using boiling water is not adequate for this purpose. (Diseases such as HIV and hepatitis can be passed on by using unsterilized needles.) Once the needle is inserted into the skin it is twisted between the acupuncturist's thumb and forefinger to spread or draw the energy from a point. The depth to which the needle is inserted can vary from just below the skin to up to 12mm (half an inch) and different sensations may be felt, such as a tingling around the area of insertion or a loss of sensation at that point. Up to 15 needles can be used but around five is generally sufficient. The length of time that they are left in varies from a few minutes to half an hour and this is dependent on a number of factors such as how the patient has reacted to previous treatment and the ailment from which he or she is suffering.

Patients can generally expect to feel an improvement after four to six sessions of therapy, the beneficial effects occurring gradually, particularly if the ailment has obvious and long-standing symptoms. Other diseases such as asthma will probably take longer before any definite improvement is felt. It is possible that some patients may not feel any improvement at all, or even feel worse after the first session and this is probably due to the energies in the body being over-stimulated. To correct this, the acupuncturist will gradually use fewer needles and for a shorter period of time. If no improvement is felt after about six to eight treatments, then it is doubtful whether acupuncture will be of any help. For general body maintenance and health, most traditional acupuncturists suggest that sessions be arranged at the time of seasonal changes.

There has been a great deal of research, particularly by the Chinese, who have produced many books detailing a high success rate for acupuncture in treating a variety of disorders. These results are, however, viewed cautiously in the West as methods of conducting clinical trials vary from East to West. Nevertheless trials have been carried out in the West and it has been discovered first consultation may last an hour, especially if detailed questioning is necessary along with the palpation.

that a pain message can be stopped from reaching the brain using acupuncture. The signal would normally travel along a nerve but it is possible to 'close a gate' on the nerve, thereby preventing the message from reaching the brain, hence preventing the perception of pain. Acupuncture is believed to work by blocking the pain signal. However, doctors stress that pain can be a warning that something is wrong or of the occurrence of a particular disease, such as cancer, that requires an orthodox remedy or method of treatment.

It has also been discovered that there are substances produced by the body that are connected with pain relief. These substances are called endorphins and encephalins, and they are natural opiates. Studies from all over the world show that acupuncture stimulates the release of these opiates into the central nervous system, thereby giving pain relief. The amount of opiates released has a direct bearing on the degree of pain relief. Acupuncture is a widely used form of anaesthesia in China where, for suitable patients, it is said to be extremely effective (90 per cent). It is used successfully during childbirth, dentistry and for operations. Orthodox doctors in the West now accept that heat treatment, massage and needles used on a sensitive part of the skin afford relief from pain caused by disease elsewhere. These areas are known as trigger points, and they are not always situated close to the organ that is affected by disease. It has been found that approximately three quarters of these trigger points are the same as the points used in Chinese acupuncture. Recent research has also shown that it is possible to find the acupuncture points by the use of electronic instruments as they register less electrical resistance than other areas of skin. As yet, no evidence has been found to substantiate the existence of meridians.

The Alexander Technique

This technique, which is based on correct posture so that the body is able to function naturally and with the minimum amount of muscular effort, was devised by Frederick Mathias Alexander (1869-1955). He was an Australian actor who found that he was losing his voice when performing but after rest his condition improved. Although he received medical help, the condition did not improve and it occurred to him that whilst acting he might be doing something that caused the problem. To see what this might be he performed his act in front of a mirror and saw what happened when he was about to speak. He experienced difficulty in breathing and lowered his head, thus making himself shorter. He realized that the strain of remembering his lines and having to project his voice, so that people furthest away in the audience would be able to hear, was causing him a great deal of stress and the way he reacted was a quite natural reflex action. In fact, even thinking about having to project his voice made the symptoms recur and from this he concluded that there must be a close connection between body and mind. He was determined to try and improve the situation and gradually, by watching and altering his stance and posture and his mental attitude to his performance on stage, matters improved. He was able to act and speak on stage and use his body in a more relaxed and natural fashion.

In 1904 Alexander travelled to London where he had decided to let others know about his method of retraining the body. He soon became very popular with other actors who appreciated the benefits of using his technique. Other public figures, such as the author Aldous Huxley, also benefited. Later he went to America, achieving considerable success and international recognition for his technique. At the age of 78 he suffered a stroke but by using his method he managed to regain the use of all his faculties-an achievement that amazed his doctors.

The Alexander technique is said to be completely harmless, encouraging an agreeable state between mind and body and is also helpful for a number of disorders such as headaches and back pain. Today, Alexander training schools can be found all over the world. A simple test to determine if people can benefit is to observe their posture. People frequently do not even stand correctly and this can encourage aches and pains if the body is unbalanced. It is incorrect to stand with round shoulders or to slouch. This often looks uncomfortable and discomfort may be felt. Sometimes people will hold themselves too erect and unbending, which again can have a bad effect. The correct posture and balance for the body needs the least muscular effort but the body will be aligned correctly. When walking one should not slouch, hold the head down or have the shoulders stooped. The head should be balanced correctly above the spine with the shoulders relaxed. It is suggested that the weight of the body should be felt being transferred from one foot to the other whilst walking.

Once a teacher has been consulted, all movements and how the body is used will be observed. Many muscles are used in everyday activities, and over the years bad habits can develop unconsciously, with stress also affecting the use of muscles. This can be demonstrated in people gripping a pen with too much force or holding the steering wheel of a car too tightly whilst driving. Muscular tension can be a serious problem affecting some people and the head, neck and back are forced out offline, which in turn leads to rounded shoulders with the head held forward and the back curved. If this situation is not altered and the body is not re-aligned correctly, the spine will become curved with a hump possibly developing. This leads to back pain and puts a strain on internal organs such as the chest and lungs.

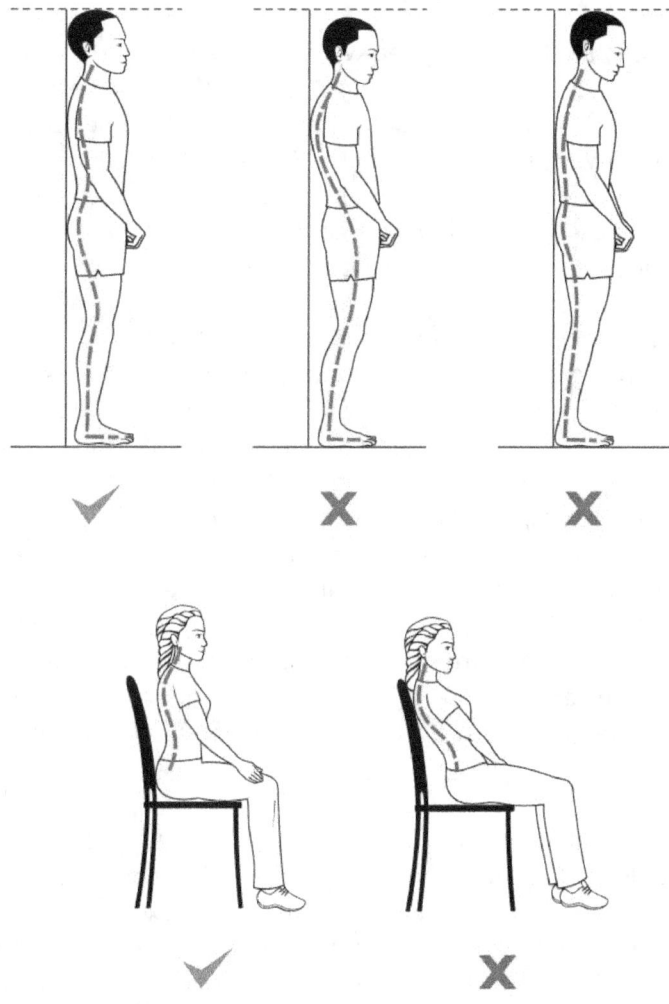

No force is used by the teacher other than some gentle manipulation to start pupils off correctly. Some teachers use light pushing methods on the back and hips, etc, while others might first ensure that the pupil is relaxed and then pull gently on the neck, which stretches the body. Any bad postures will be corrected by the teacher and the pupil will be shown how best to alter this so that muscles will be used most effectively and with the least effort.

Any manipulation that is used will be to ease the body into a more relaxed and natural position. It is helpful to be completely aware of using the technique not only on the body but also with the mind. With frequent use of the Alexander technique for posture and the release of tension, the muscles and the body should be used correctly with a consequent improvement in, for example, the manner of walking and sitting.

The length of time for each lesson can vary from about half an hour to three quarters of an hour and the number of lessons is usually between 10 and 30, by which time pupils should have gained sufficient knowledge to continue practising the technique by themselves. Once a person has learned how to improve posture, it will be found that he or she is taller and carrying the body in a more upright manner. The technique has been found to be of benefit to dancers, athletes and those having to speak in public. Other disorders claimed to have been treated successfully are depressive states, headaches caused by tension, anxiety, asthma, hypertension, respiratory problems, colitis, osteoarthritis and rheumatoid arthritis, sciatica and peptic ulcer.

The Alexander technique is recommended for all ages and types of people as their overall quality of life, both mental and physical, can be improved. People can learn how to resist stress and one eminent professor experienced a great improvement in a variety of ways: in quality of sleep; lessening of high blood pressure and improved mental awareness. He even found that his ability to play a musical instrument had improved.

The Alexander technique can be applied to two positions adopted every day, namely sitting in a chair and sitting at a desk. To be seated in the correct manner the head should be comfortably balanced, with no tension in the shoulders, and a small gap between the knees (if legs are crossed the spine and pelvis become out of line or twisted) and the soles of the feet should be flat on the floor. It is incorrect to sit with the head lowered and the shoulders slumped forward because the stomach becomes restricted and breathing may also be affected. On the other hand, it is also incorrect to hold the body in a stiff and erect position.

To sit correctly while working at a table, the body should be held upright but in a relaxed manner with any bending movement coming from the hips and with the seat flat on the chair. If writing, the pen should be held lightly and if using a computer one should ensure that the arms are relaxed and feel comfortable. The chair should be set at a comfortable height with regard to the level of the desk. It is incorrect to lean forward over a desk because this hampers breathing, or to hold the arms in a tense, tight manner.

There has been some scientific research carried out that concurs with the beliefs that Alexander formed, such as the relationship between mind and body (the thought of doing an action actually triggering a physical reaction or tension). Today, doctors do not have any opposition to the Alexander technique and may recommend
it on occasions.

Aromatherapy

Aromatherapy is a method of healing using very concentrated essential oils that are often highly aromatic and are extracted from plants. Constituents of the oils confer the characteristic perfume or odour given off by a particular plant. Essential oils help the plant in some way to complete its cycle of growth and reproduction.

For example, some oils may attract insects for the purpose of pollination; others may render it distasteful as a source of food. Any part of a plant-the stems, leaves, flowers, fruits, seeds, roots or bark-may produce essential oils or essences but often only in minute amounts. Different parts of the same plant may produce their own form of oil. An example of this is the orange, which produces oils with different properties in the flowers, fruits and leaves.

The therapeutic and medicinal properties of plant extracts have long been recognized and their use dates back to earliest times. Art and writings from the ancient civilizations of Egypt, China and Persia show that plant essences were used and valued by priests, physicians and healers. Plant essences have been used throughout the ages for healing-in incense for religious rituals, in perfumes and embalming ointments and for culinary purposes. There are many Biblical references that give an insight into the uses of plant oils and the high value that was attached to them. Throughout the course of human history the healing properties of plants and their essential oils has been recognized and most people probably had some knowledge about their use. It was only in more recent times, with the great developments in science and orthodox medicine, particularly the manufacture of antibiotics and synthetic drugs, that knowledge and interest in the older methods of healing declined. However, in the last few years there has been a great rekindling of interest in the practice of aromatherapy with many people turning to this form of treatment.

Extraction of essential oils

Since any part of a plant may produce essential oils, the method of extraction depends upon the site and accessibility of the essence in each particular case. The oils are produced by special minute cells or glands and are released naturally by the plant in small amounts over a prolonged period of time when needed. In order to harvest the oils in appreciable amounts, it is usually necessary to collect a large quantity of the part of the plant needed and to subject the material to a process that causes the oil glands to burst. One of the most common methods is steam distillation.

The plant material is paced tightly into a press or still and steamed at a high temperature. This causes the oil glands to burst and the essential oil vaporises into the steam. This is then cooled to separate the oil from the water. Sometimes water is used for distillation rather than steam. Another method involved dissolving the plant material in a solvent or alcohol and is called solvent extraction. This involves placing the material in a centrifuge, which rotates at high speed, and then extracting the essential oils by means of a low temperature distillation process. Substances obtained in this way may be called resins or absolutes. A further method is called maceration in which the plant is soaked in hot oil. The plant cells collapse and release their essential oils, and the whole mixture is then separated and purified by a process called defleurage. If fat is used instead of oil, the process is called enfleurage. These methods produce a purer oil that is usually more expensive than one obtained by distillation. The essential oils used in aromatherapy tend to be costly as vast quantities of plant material are required to produce them and the methods used are complex and costly.

Storage and use of essential oils

Essential oils are highly concentrated, volatile and aromatic. They readily evaporate and change and deteriorate if exposed to light, heat and air. Hence pure oils need to be stored carefully in brown glass bottles at a moderate temperature away from direct light. They can be stored for one or two years in this way. For most purposes in aromatherapy, essential oils are used in a dilute form, being added either to water or to another oil, called the base or carrier. The base is often a vegetable oil such as olive or safflower, which both have nutrient and beneficial properties. An essential/carrier oil mixture has a short useful life of two or three months and so they are usually mixed at the time of use and in small amounts.

Techniques used in aromatherapy

There are four techniques used in aromatherapy and these are *massage, bathing, inhalation* and *compresses*.

Massage is the most familiar method of treatment associated with aromatherapy. Essential oils are able to penetrate through the skin and are taken into the body, exerting healing and beneficial influences on internal tissues and organs. The oils used for massage are first diluted by being mixed with a base and should never be applied directly to the skin in their pure form in case of an adverse allergic reaction.

Bathing most people have experienced the benefits of relaxing in a hot bath to which a proprietary perfumed preparation has been added. Most of these preparations contain essential oils used in aromatherapy. The addition of a number of drops of an essential oil to the bath water can have great beneficial effects. It is soothing and relaxing, easing aches and pains, and can also have a stimulating effect, banishing tiredness and restoring energy, depending upon the type of oil that is used. In addition, there is the added benefit of inhaling the vapours of the oil as they evaporate from the hot water.

Inhalation is thought to be the most direct and rapid means of treatment. This is because the molecules of the volatile essential oil act directly on the olfactory organs and are immediately perceived by the brain. A popular method is the time-honoured one of *steam inhalation,* in which a few drops of essential oil are added to hot water in a bowl. The person sits with his or her face above the mixture and covers the head, face and bowl with a towel so that the vapours do not escape. This can be repeated up to three times a day but should not be undertaken by people suffering from asthma. Some essential oils can be applied directly to a handkerchief or onto a pillow and the vapours inhaled in this way.

Compresses to prepare a compress in aromatherapy, a few drops of essential oil are added to a proportion of hot or cold water and then a cloth is soaked in the mixture. The cloth is wrung out, (although kept fairly wet) and applied to the painful part, and is tied in place with Clingfilm and a bandage. The compress needs to be left in place for two hours before being changed. Usually, hot compresses are applied to chronic persistent pain. For conditions in which there is heat, inflammation, swelling and fever, a cold compress is generally indicated.

Essential oils may also be diluted with water and used in hand and foot baths if only a small area of the body needs to be treated. Some are appropriate for use as gargles and mouth washes, and are helpful in clearing up infections such as mouth ulcers. However, they should never be swallowed. Essential oils can be used effectively in the home by adding a few drops into a bowl of water or potpourri and leaving to stand in a room.

Mode of action of essential oils

Although the subject of a great deal of research, there is a lack of knowledge about how essential oils work in the body to produce their therapeutic effects. It is known that individual essential oils possess antiseptic, antibiotic, sedative, tonic and stimulating properties, and it is believed that they act in harmony with the natural defences of the body such as the immune system. Some oils, such as eucalyptus and rosemary, act as natural decongestants whereas others, such as sage, have a beneficial effect upon the circulation.

Conditions that may benefit from aromatherapy

A wide range of conditions and disorders may benefit from aromatherapy and it is considered to be a gentle treatment suitable for all age groups. It is especially beneficial for long-term chronic conditions, and the use of essential oils is believed by therapists to prevent the development of some illnesses. Conditions that may be relieved by aromatherapy include painful limbs, muscles and joints due to arthritic or rheumatic disorders, respiratory complaints, digestive disorders, skin conditions, throat and mouth infections, urinary tract infections and problems affecting the hair and scalp. Also, period pains, bums, insect bites and stings, headaches, high blood pressure, feverishness, menopausal symptoms, poor circulation and gout can benefit from aromatherapy. Aromatherapy is of great benefit in relieving stress and stress-related symptoms such as anxiety, insomnia and depression.

Many of the essential oils can be safely used at home and the basic techniques of use can soon be mastered. However, some should only be used by a trained aromatherapist and others must be avoided in certain conditions such as pregnancy. In some circumstances, massage is not considered to be advisable. It is wise to seek medical advice in the event of doubt or if the ailment is more than a minor one.

Consulting a professional aromatherapist

Aromatherapy is a holistic approach to healing hence the practitioner endeavours to build up a complete picture of the patient and his or her lifestyle, nature and family circumstances, as well as noting the symptoms which need to be to be treated. Depending upon the picture that is obtained, the aromatherapist decides upon the essential oil or oils that are most suitable and likely to prove most helpful in the circumstances that prevail. The aromatherapist has a wide ranging knowledge and experience upon which to draw. Many oils can be blended together for an enhanced effect and this is called a 'synergistic blend'. Many aromatherapists offer a massage and/or instruction on the use of the selected oils at home.

Examples of some essential oils

Basil is now grown in many countries of the world although it originates from Africa. The herb has a long history of medicinal and culinary use, and was familiar to the Ancient Egyptian and Greek civilizations. Basil is sacred in the Hindu religion and has many medicinal uses in India and other Eastern countries. The whole plant is subjected to a process of steam distillation to obtain the essential oil used in aromatherapy. Basil has a refreshing, invigorating effect and also has antiseptic properties. It is used in massage, inhalation and baths, and can help to relieve the symptoms of tiredness, colds and respiratory disorders, indigestion and digestive problems, and minor skin wounds and rashes. It can help to alleviate the symptoms of depression although it has a depressive effect if used to excess.

Bergamot oil of bergamot is obtained from a plant that is a native species of some Asian and Eastern countries. The oil was first used and traded in Italy and derives its name from the northern city of Bergamo. In Italian medicine, it was popular as a remedy for feverish illnesses and to expel intestinal worms. It has also been used in cosmetics and perfumes, as the flavouring of Earl Grey tea, and in other foods. The oil is squeezed from the peel of the fruits for use in aromatherapy. It has refreshing, soothing and antiseptic properties, and may be combined with eucalyptus to enhance its effects. It can be used in massage, inhalation and baths, and helps to relieve painful or itchy skin conditions such as psoriasis. It is also used to treat cold sores, mouth and throat infections, shingles, ulcers and symptoms of depression and tiredness.

Eucalyptus is a native species of Australia and Tasmania but is now grown in many countries throughout the world. The planthas a characteristic pungent odour, and the oil obtained from it has disinfectant and antiseptic properties, clears the nasal passages and acts as a painkiller. The leaves and twigs are subjected to a process of steam distillation in order to obtain the essential oil used in aromatherapy. The diluted oil is used for muscular and rheumatic aches and pains, skin disorders such as ringworm, insect bites, headaches and neuralgia, shingles, respiratory and bronchitic infections and fevers. Eucalyptus is used in many household products and in remedies for coughs and colds.

Juniper is a native species of many northern countries and has a long history of medicinal use. It has stimulant, tonic and antiseptic properties with beneficial effects on the skin and the digestive and reproductive organs. It is used to relieve the symptoms of dermatitis, eczema, spots, and dry, sore and chafed skin. Also, it is helpful in the relief of gout and painful rheumatoid arthritis. It is beneficial in the treatment of stress and sleeplessness. In cases of debility, it helps by acting as a tonic for the digestion and boosting the appetite. It can be used in massage, baths and inhalation, and is a useful treatment for cystitis, haemorrhoids (piles) and menstrual problems. Juniper is also used in veterinary medicine and as an ingredient in some toiletries.

Lavender the highly perfumed lavender is a native species of the Mediterranean but has long been popular as a garden plant in Britain, America and many other countries. It has antiseptic, tonic and relaxing properties, and the essential oil used in aromatherapy is obtained by subjecting the flowers to a process of steam distillation. It is considered to be one of the safest preparations and is used in the treatment of a wide range of disorders. These include minor skin wounds and burns, insect bites, indigestion and digestive problems, muscle pains and strains, cystitis, period pains and premenstrual symptoms, headaches, depression and stress. Lavender is also widely used in perfumes, toiletries and household preparations.

Peppermint is a native plant of Europe with a long history of medicinal use dating back to the ancient civilizations of Egypt, Greece and Rome. Oil of peppermint is obtained by subjecting the flowering parts of the plant to a process of steam distillation. The essential oil of peppermint has a calming effect on the digestive tract and is excellent for the relief of indigestion, colic-type pains, nausea, travel and morning sickness. It is cooling and refreshing, and useful in the treatment of colds, respiratory symptoms and headaches. Peppermint is widely used in remedies for colds and indigestion, as a food flavouring, especially in confectionery, and in toothpaste.

Sage is a native plant of the northern coastal regions of the Mediterranean and has a long history of medicinal and culinary use dating back to the ancient civilizations of Greece and Rome. The essential oil used in aromatherapy is obtained by subjecting the dried leaves to a process of steam distillation. Sage has a stimulating effect upon the circulation and also has tonic, antiseptic, expectorant (when inhaled) and cooling properties. It is used to improve poor circulation, for sore throats, colds and viral infections, bronchitic and catarrhal complaints, rheumatism, arthritic pains, joint sprains and strains, mouth infections and headaches. Sage is widely used as a flavouring in foods and in some household preparations and toiletries.

Ylang ylang is a native species of the Far Eastern islands of Indonesia, the Philippines, Java and Madagascar. To obtain the essential oil used in aromatherapy, the flowers are subjected to a
process of steam distillation. The oil has antiseptic and relaxing properties and is also believed to be an aphrodisiac. It has a calming effect on the heart-beat rate and can be used to relieve palpitations, tachycardia, hypertension (raised blood pressure), depression and shock. It has a tonic effect upon the skin and is beneficial in the treatment of nervous complaints. Ylang ylang is used in perfumes and toiletries and as a flavouring in the food industry.

Auricular Therapy

A method of healing using stimulation of different acupuncture points on the surface of the ear. Auricular therapists claim that there are over two hundred points on the ear that are connected to a particular organ, tissue or part of the body. If a disorder is present, its corresponding point on the ear may be sensitive or tender to touch and pressure, or there may even be some kind of physical sign such as a mark, spot or lump. Stimulation of the ear is carried out by means of acupuncture needles, or minute electric currents or a laser beam may be used.

It is claimed that auricular therapy is helpful in the treatment of various chronic conditions such as rheumatism and arthritis and also problems of addiction. During a first consultation, the auricular therapist obtains a detailed picture of the patient's state of health, lifestyle and family background. A physical examination of the ears is carried out and any distinguishing features are recorded. The therapist passes a probe over the surface of the ear to find any sensitive points that indicate the areas requiring treatment.

The practice of manipulating needles in the ear to cure diseases in other parts of the body is a very ancient one. It has been used for many hundreds of years in some Eastern and Mediterranean countries and in China. Although the method of action is not understood, auricular therapy is becoming increasingly popular.

Autogenic Training

Autogenic training is a form of therapy that seeks to teach the patient to relax, thereby relieving stress. This is achieved by the patient learning a series of six basic exercises that can be undertaken either lying flat on the back, sitting in an armchair or sitting towards the edge of a chair with the head bent forwards and the chin on the chest. The six exercises concentrate on (a) breathing and respiration (b) heartbeat (c) the forehead to induce a feeling of coolness (d) the lower abdomen and stomach to induce a feeling of warmth (e) the arms and legs to induce a feeling of warmth (f) the neck, shoulders, arms and legs to induce a feeling of heaviness.

It is now well established that a number of illnesses and disorders are related to, or made worse by, stress. By learning the techniques and exercises of autogenic training, the person is able to achieve a state of relaxation and tranquillity, sleeps better and generally has more energy and a greater feeling of wellbeing. Autogenic training is taught at group sessions involving a small number of people (about six is usual).

Patients with a variety of disorders may benefit from autogenic training, which can also help people who feel under stress without particular physical symptoms. Illnesses that may be helped include irritable bowel syndrome, digestive disorders, muscular aches and cramps, ulcers, headaches and high blood pressure. Also, anxieties, fears and phobias, insomnia and some other psychological
illnesses. This form of therapy can benefit people of all age groups, although it is considered that children under the age of six may not be able to understand the training. Therapists in autogenic training usually hold medical or nursing qualifications and expect to obtain a full picture of the patient's state of health before treatment begins.

Ayurvedic Medicine

A holistic approach to health care that, alongside orthodox medicine, is a major form of therapy in India and is gaining an increasing number of followers in Western Countries. A great deal of emphasis is placed on preventative measures to maintain good health. Hence the practitioner in Ayurvedic Medicine obtains a detailed picture of all aspects of the patient's life and has frequent consultations with the person. If any aspect of the patient's life undergoes a change the practitioner may advise some form of treatment to prevent any problems from occurring. Methods of treatment include a great variety of medicines that are derived from plant and mineral sources, meditation, yoga and other exercises, religious ceremonies, water and steam baths, massage and specially planned diets.

In the Ayurvedic philosophy, everything in life is held to be controlled by three forces which are called pitta, vata and kapha. Pitta is said to be like the sun, a great source of energy and in control of all metabolic processes and bodily functions. Vata resembles the wind, which is a continual source of movement and controls the workings of the brain and nervous system. Kapha is like the moon and its tidal influences, and controls the fluids of the body and the growth and regeneration of cells. Also, in Ayurvedic medicine all disorders are grouped into four broad categories (although a holistic approach is still maintained). These are: (1) Mental, covering disorders or symptoms with an emotional basis especially the stronger feelings such as jealousy, fears and phobias, hatred, rage and depression; (2) physical, covering most illnesses and internal disorders; (3) accidental, covering illnesses and disorders that are caused by some form of external trauma; (4) natural disorders or symptoms that are particularly associated with certain ages or stages in life.

In Ayurvedic medicine it is believed that good health results from the three forces of pitta, kapha and vata being balanced and in harmony with one another. If one force becomes relatively stronger or weaker than the others, then disorder arises causing symptoms of illness. A person 'inherits' his or her own particular balance of forces at the moment of conception. Imbalance in any of the three forces may arise as a result of stressful life events or due to a lack of care in maintaining the balance.

There are an increasing number of practitioners of Ayurvedic medicine in Great Britain. Many believe that its greatest strength lies in its emphasis on the maintenance of good health and prevention of problems or illnesses before they arise. The fact that the physician and the patient need to have a close working relationship no doubt provides reassurance for many of the followers of Ayurvedic medicine.

Chiropractic

The word chiropractic originates from two Greek words kheir, which means 'hand', and praktikos, which means 'practical'. A school of chiropractic was established in about 1895 by a healer called Daniel Palmer (1845-1913). He was able to cure a man's deafness that had occurred when he bent down and felt a bone click. Upon examination Palmer discovered that some bones of the man's spine had become displaced. After successful manipulation the man regained his hearing. Palmer formed the opinion that if there was any displacement in the skeleton this could affect the function of nerves, either increasing or decreasing their action and thereby resulting in a malfunction i.e. a disease.

Chiropractic is used to relieve pain by manipulation and to correct any problems that are present in joints and muscles but especially the spine. Like osteopathy, no use is made of surgery or drugs. If there are any spinal disorders they can cause widespread problems elsewhere in the body such as the hip, leg or arm and can also initiate lumbago, sciatica, a slipped disc or other back problems. It is even possible that spinal problems can result in seemingly unrelated problems such as catarrh, migraine, asthma, constipation, stress, etc. However, the majority of a chiropractor's patients suffer mainly from neck and back pain. People suffering from whiplash injuries sustained in car accidents commonly seek the help of a chiropractor. The whiplash effect is caused when the head is violently wrenched either forwards or backwards at the time of impact.

Another common problem that chiropractors treat is headaches, and it is often the case that tension is the underlying cause as it makes the neck muscles contract. Athletes can also obtain relief from injuries such as tennis elbow, pulled muscles, injured ligaments and sprains, etc. As well as the normal methods of manipulating joints, the chiropractor may decide it is necessary to use applications of ice or heat to relieve the injury.

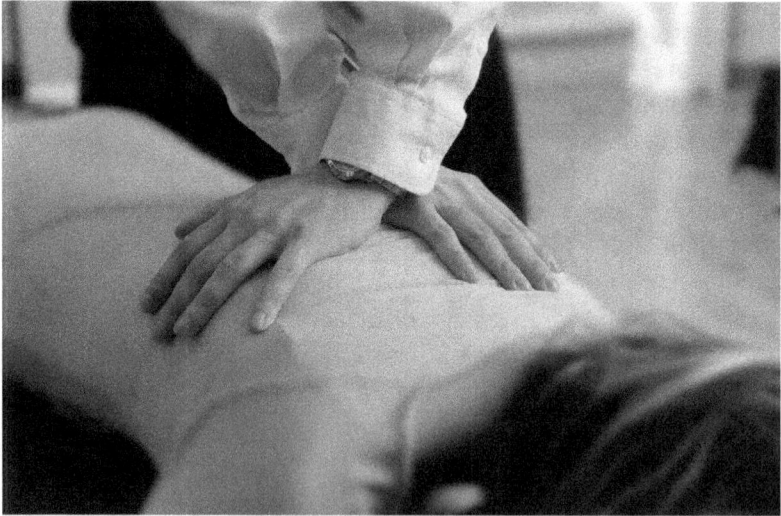

Children can also benefit from treatment by a chiropractor, as there may be some slight accident that occurs in their early years that can reappear in adult life in the form of back pain. It can easily happen, for example, when a child learns to walk and bumps into furniture, or when a baby falls out of a cot. This could result in some damage to the spine that will show only in adult life when a person experiences back pain. At birth, a baby's neck may be injured or the spine may be strained if the use of forceps is necessary, and this can result in headaches and neck problems as he or she grows to maturity. This early type of injury could also account for what is known as 'growing pains', when the real problem is actually damage that has been done to the bones or muscles. If a parent has any worries it is best to consult a doctor and it is possible that the child will be recommended to see a qualified chiropractor. To avoid any problems in adult life, chiropractors recommend that children have occasional examinations to detect any damage or displacement in bones and muscles.

As well as babies and children, adults of all ages can benefit from chiropractic. There are some people who regularly take painkillers for painful joints or back pain, but this does not deal with the root cause of the pain, only the symptoms that are produced. It is claimed that chiropractic could be of considerable help in giving treatment to these people. Many pregnant women experience backache at some stage during their pregnancy because of the extra weight that is placed on the spine, and they also may find it difficult keeping their balance. At the time of giving birth, changes take place in the pelvis and joints at the bottom of the spine and this can be a cause of back pain. Lifting and carrying babies, if not done correctly, can also damage the spine and thereby make the back painful.

It is essential that any chiropractor is fully qualified and registered with the relevant professional association. At the initial visit, a patient will be for asked details of his or her case history, including the present problem, and during the examination painful and tender areas will be noted and joints will be checked to see whether they are functioning correctly or not. X-rays are frequently used by chiropractors as these help them to make a detailed diagnosis since they can show signs of bone disease, fractures or arthritis as well as the spine's condition. After the initial visit, any treatment will normally begin as soon as the patient has been informed of the chiropractor's diagnosis. If it has been decided that chiropractic therapy will not be of any benefit, the patient will be advised accordingly.

For treatment, underwear and/or a robe will be worn, and the patient will either lie, sit or stand on a specially designed couch. Chiropractors use their hands in a skilful way to effect the different manipulative techniques. If it is decided that manipulation is necessary to treat a painful lumbar joint, the patient will need to lie on his or her side. The upper and lower spine will then be rotated manually but in opposite ways. This manipulation will have the effect of partially locking the joint that is being treated, and the upper leg is usually flexed to aid the procedure.

The vertebra that is immediately below or above the joint will then be felt by the chiropractor, and the combination of how the patient is lying, coupled with gentle pressure applied by the chiropractor's hand, will move the joint to its furthest extent of normal movement. There will then be a very quick push applied on the vertebra, which results in its movement being extended further than normal, ensuring that full use of the joint is regained. This is due to the muscles that surround the joint being suddenly stretched, which has the effect of relaxing the muscles of the spine that work upon the joint. This alteration should cause the joint to be able to be used more naturally and should not be a painful procedure. There can be a variety of effects felt after treatment-some patients may feel sore or stiff, or may ache some time after the treatment, while others will experience the lifting of pain at once. In some cases there may be a need for multiple treatments, perhaps four or more, before improvement is felt. On the whole, problems that have been troubling a patient for a considerable time (chronic) will need more therapy than anything that occurs quickly and is very painful (acute).

Although there is only quite a small number of chiropractors - yet this numbers is increasing-there is a degree of contact and liaison between them and doctors. It is generally accepted that chiropractic is an effective remedy for bone and muscular problems, and the majority of doctors would be happy to accept a chiropractor's diagnosis and treatment, although the treatment of any general diseases, such as diabetes or asthma, would not be viewed in the same manner.

Colour Therapy

Colour therapy uses coloured light to treat disease and disorder and to help restore good health. It is well known that human beings respond to coloured light and are affected in different ways by rays of various wavelengths. This even occurs in people who are blind, so the human body is able to respond in subtle ways to electromagnetic radiation. Colour therapists believe that each individual receives and absorbs electromagnetic radiation from the sun and emits it in a unique 'aura' -a pattern of colours peculiar to that person. It is believed that the aura can be recorded on film by a photographic technique known as Kirlian photography. If disease is present, this manifests itself as a disturbance of the vibrations that form the aura, giving a distorted pattern. During a consultation, a colour therapist pays particular attention to the patient's spine as each individual vertebra is believed to reflect the condition of a particular part of the body. Hence the aura from each vertebra is believed to indicate the health of its corresponding body part. Each vertebra is believed to be related to one of the eight colours of the visible spectrum. The eight colours are repeated in their usual sequence from the top to the base of the spine.

The treatment consists of bathing the body in coloured light. With appropriate colours being decided upon by the therapist. Usually one main colour is used along with a complementary one, and the light is emitted in irregular bursts. Treatment sessions last for a little less than twenty minutes and are continued for at least seven weeks. The aim is to restore the natural balance in the pattern of the aura. A therapist also advises on the use of colours in the home and of clothes and soft furnishings, etc.

In orthodox medicine it is accepted that colours exert subtle influences on people, especially affecting their state of mind and psychological wellbeing. Colour therapy may well aid healing, but there is no scientific evidence to explain the way in which this might work.

Dance Movement Therapy

Dance movement therapy is aimed at helping people to resolve deep-seated problems by communicating with, and relating to others through the medium of physical movements and dance. The ability to express deep inner feelings in 'body language' and physical movements is innate in human beings. Young children express themselves freely in this way and without inhibition, and dancing would appear to be common to all past and present races and tribes of people. However, in modern industrial societies, many people find themselves unable to communicate their problems and fears either verbally or physically and may repress them to such an extent that they become ill. Dance movement therapy aims to help people to explore, recognize and come to terms with feelings and problems that they usually repress, and to communicate them to others. This therapy can help emotional, psychological and stress related disorders, anxiety and depression, addiction, problems related to physical or sexual abuse, and learning disabilities. Children are often very responsive to this therapy and may have behavioural or intellectual problems, autism or other mental and physical disabilities.

People of any age can take part in dance movement therapy as the aim is to explore gently physical movements that are within each person's capabilities. The therapist may suggest movements, but hopes to encourage patients to learn to take the initiative. Eventually some groups learn to talk over feelings and problems that have emerged through taking part and are better able to resolve them.

Dance therapy sessions are organized in some hospitals and 'drop-in' and day-care centres. This form of therapy is regarded as particularly beneficial for people suffering from a number of disorders, particularly those with psychological and emotional problems or who are intellectually disadvantaged.

Do-in

Do-in (pronounced doe-in) is another ancient type of massage that originated in China. It is a technique of self-massage and, as in other forms of alternative therapy, it is believed that there is a flow of energy throughout the body that travels along 'meridians' and that each of these is connected to a vital organ such as the lungs, liver and heart. Do-in has a connection with shiatsu, and people of any age can participate, the only stipulation being that they are active and not out of condition. Clothing should not be tight or restrictive and adequate space is needed to perform the exercises.

If do-in is to be used as an invigorating form of massage, then the best time of day is as soon as possible after rising, but not after breakfast. After meals are the only times when do-in is to be avoided. It is generally recommended that people wishing to practise do-in should first go to classes where it is being taught, so that when the exercises are done at home they are performed correctly. It is claimed that the use of do-in is preventive in nature since the vital organs are strengthened and therefore maintained in a healthy state. As in massage, this is a deterrent to the nervous tension, strain and stress experienced by many people in modern life. It is also claimed to be beneficial for people suffering from arthritis and rheumatism.

Before starting, it is best to do some warming-up exercises so that the body is not stiff. Begin by sitting on the ground with the knees up, grasp the knees and begin a rocking motion forwards and backwards. Then sit up, again on the floor, position the legs as if to sit cross-legged but put the soles of the feet touching each other. Hold the toes for a short time. These two exercises should help to make the body more supple.

For the spleen meridian exercise, which is connected with the stomach, stand as near as possible in front of a wall. Place one hand palm downwards high up the wall so that there is a good stretching action and with the other hand grasp the foot that is opposite to the raised arm. Then the neck and head should be stretched backwards, away from the wall. Maintain this stretched position and inhale and exhale deeply twice and then relax. Repeat the procedure using the other arm and leg.

For the bladder meridian exercise, and thereby the kidneys, sit on the floor with the legs straight out in front and ensure that the toes are tensed upright. The arms should then be stretched above the head and a breath taken. After breathing out, bend forwards from the shoulders with the arms in front and hold the toes. Maintain this for the length of time it takes to breathe in and out three times. Repeat the whole procedure again.

To do the exercise for the pericardium meridian, which affects the circulation, sit on the floor with feet touching, but one behind the other, ensuring that the hands are crossed and touching opposite knees. Grasp the knees and incline the body forwards with the aim of pushing the knees downwards on to the floor. Do this exercise again but with the hands on opposite knees and the other foot on the outside.

Using the exercise that strengthens the large intestine meridian and in turn the lungs, stand upright with the feet apart. Link the thumbs behind the back and then inhale. Exhale and at the same time place the arms outwards and upwards behind the back. To complete the exercise. lean forwards from the hips and then stand upright.

To strengthen the liver by stimulating the gall bladder meridian, sit upright on the floor with the legs the maximum distance apart. Then inhale, passing the arms along the length of the right leg so that the base of the foot can be held. There should be no movement of the buttocks off the floor. Maintain this stretched position while breathing deeply twice. Repeat the exercise using the other leg.

After all exercises have been accomplished, lie flat out on the floor with the legs apart and the arms stretched at the sides, palms uppermost. Then lift the head so that the feet can be seen and then put the head back on the floor again. The head and body should then be shaken so that the legs, arms and neck are loosened. To complete the relaxation, the eyes should be closed and the person should lie quietly for a few minutes.

Herbal Medicine

History of the use of herbal remedies

The medicinal use of herbs is said to be as old as mankind itself. In early civilizations, food and medicine were linked and many plants were eaten for their health-giving properties. In ancient

Egypt, the slave workers were given a daily ration of garlic to help fight off the many fevers and infections that were common at that time. The first written records of herbs and their beneficial properties were compiled by the ancient Egyptians. Most of our knowledge and use of herbs can be traced back to the Egyptian priests who also practised herbal medicine. Records dating back to 1500 ne listed medicinal herbs, including caraway and cinnamon.

The ancient Greeks and Romans also carried out herbal medicine, and as they invaded new lands their doctors encountered new herbs and introduced herbs such as rosemary or lavender into new areas. Other cultures with a history of herbal medicine are the Chinese and the Indians. In Britain, the use of herbs developed along with the establishment of monasteries around the country, each of which had its own herb garden for use in treating both the monks and the local people. In some areas, particularly Wales and Scotland, Druids and other Celtic healers are thought to have had an oral tradition of herbalism, where medicine was mixed with religion and ritual.

Over time, these healers and their knowledge led to the writing of the first 'herbals', which rapidly rose in importance and distribution upon the advent of the printing press in the 15th century. John Parkinson of London wrote a herbal around 1630, listing useful plants. Many herbalists set up their own apothecary shops, including the famous Nicholas Culpepper (1616-1654) whose most famous work is *The Complete Herbal and English Physician, Enlarged,* published in 1649. Then in 1812, Henry Potter started a business supplying herbs and dealing in leeches. By this time a huge amount of traditional knowledge and folklore on medicinal herbs was available from Britain, Europe, the Middle East, Asia and the Americas. This promoted Potter to write *Potters Encyclopaedia of Botanical Drugs and Preparations,* which is still published today.

It was in this period that scientifically inspired conventional medicine rose in popularity, sending herbal medicine into a decline. In rural areas, herbal medicine continued to thrive in local folklore, traditions and practices. In 1864 the National Association (later Institute) of Medical Herbalists was established, to organize training of herbal medicine practitioners and to maintain standards of practice. From 1864 until the early part of this century, the Institute fought attempts to ban herbal medicine and over time public interest in herbal medicine has increased, particularly over the last 20 years. This move away from synthetic drugs is partly due to possible side effects, bad publicity, and, in some instances, a mistrust of the medical and pharmacological industries.

The more natural appearance of herbal remedies has led to its growing support and popularity. Herbs from America have been incorporated with common remedies and scientific research into herbs and their active ingredients has confirmed their healing power and enlarged the range of medicinal herbs used today.

Herbal medicine can be viewed as the precursor of modern pharmacology, but today it continues as an effective and more natural method of treating and preventing illness. Globally, herbal medicine is three to four times more commonly practised than conventional medicine.

Forms of herbal preparations

capsule this is a gelatine container for swallowing and holding oils or balsams that would otherwise be difficult to administer due to their unpleasant taste or smell. It is used for cod liver oil and castor oil.

decoction this is prepared using cut, bruised or ground bark and roots placed into a stainless steel or enamel pan (not aluminium) with cold water poured on. The mixture is boiled for 20-30 minutes, cooled and strained. It is best drunk when warm.

herbal dressing this may be a compress or poultice. A compress is made of cloth or cotton wool soaked in cold or warm herbal decoctions or infusions while a poultice can be made with fresh or dried herbs. Bruised fresh herbs are applied directly to the affected area and dried herbs are made into a paste with water and placed on gauze on the required area. Both dressings are very effective in easing pain, swelling and inflammation of the skin and tissues.

infusion this liquid is made from ground or bruised roots, bark, herbs or seeds, by pouring boiling water onto the herb and leaving it to stand for 10-30 minutes, possibly stirring the mixture occasionally. The resultant liquid is strained and used. Cold infusions may be made if the active principles are yielded from the herb without heat. Today, infusions may be packaged into teabags for convenience.

liquid extract this preparation, if correctly made, is the most concentrated fluid form in which herbal drugs may be obtained and, as such, is very popular and convenient. Each herb is treated by various means dependent upon the individual properties of the herb, e.g. cold percolation, high pressure, evaporation by heat in a vacuum. These extracts are commonly held in a household stock of domestic remedies.

pessary similar to suppositories, but it is used in female complaints to apply a preparation to the walls of the vagina and cervix.

pill probably the best known and most widely used herbal preparation. It is normally composed of concentrated extracts and alkaloids, in combination with active crude drugs. The pill may be coated with sugar or another pleasant-tasting substance that is readily soluble in the stomach.

solid extract this type of preparation is prepared by evaporating the fresh juices or strong infusions of herbal drugs to the consistency of honey. It may also be prepared from an alcoholic tincture base. It is used mainly to produce pills, plasters, ointments and compressed tablets.

suppository this preparation is a small cone of a convenient and easily soluble base with herbal extracts added, which is used to apply medicines to the rectum. It is very effective in the treatment of piles, cancers, etc.

tablet this is made by compressing drugs into a small compass. It is more easily administered and has a quicker action as it dissolves more rapidly in the stomach.

tincture this is the most prescribed form of herbal medicine. It is based on alcohol and, as such, removes certain active principles from herbs that will not dissolve in water, or in the presence of heat. The tincture produced is long-lasting, highly concentrated and only needs to be taken in small doses for beneficial effects. The ground or chopped dried herb is placed in a container with 40 per cent alcohol such as gin or vodka and left for two weeks. The tincture is then decanted into a dark bottle and sealed before use.

Medical terms

In homoeopathy and herbal treatments there are numerous terms used. Listed below are some of the more common terms likely to be encountered in the example herbs provided in this section.

alterative a term given to a substance that speeds up the renewal of the tissues, so that they can carry out their functions more effectively.

anodyne a drug that eases and soothes pain.

anthelmintic a substance that causes the death or expulsion of parasitic worms.

antiperiodic a drug that prevents the return of recurring diseases, e.g. malaria.

antiscorbutic a substance that prevents scurvy and contains necessary vitamins, e.g. vitamin C.

antiseptic a substance that prevents the growth of disease-causing microorganisms, e.g. bacteria, without causing damage to living tissue. It is applied to wounds to cleanse them and prevent infection.

antispasmodic a drug that diminishes muscle spasms.

aperient a medicine that produces a natural movement of the bowel.

aphrodisiac a compound that excites the sexual organs.

aromatic a substance that has an aroma.

astringent a substance that causes cells to contract by losing proteins from their surface. This causes localized contraction of blood vessels and tissues.

balsamic a substance that contains resins and benzoic acid and that is used to alleviate colds and abrasions.

bitter a drug that is bitter-tasting and is used to stimulate the appetite.

cardiac compounds that have some effect on the heart.

carminative a preparation to relieve flatulence and griping.

cathartic a compound that produces an evacuation of the bowels.

cooling a substance that reduces the temperature and cools the skin.

demulcent a substance that soothes and protects the alimentary canal.

deobstruent a compound that is said to clear obstructions, and open the natural passages of the body.

detergent a substance that has a cleansing action, either internally or on the skin.

diaphoretic a term given to drugs that promote perspiration.

diuretics applied to substances that stimulate the kidneys and increase urine and solute production.

emetic a drug that induces vomiting.

emmenagogue a compound that is able to excite the menstrual discharge.

emollient a substance that softens or soothes the skin.

expectorant a group of drugs that are taken to help in the removal of secretions from the lungs, bronchi and trachea.

febrifuge a substance that reduces fever.

galactogogue an agent that stimulates the production of breast milk or increases milk flow.

hydrogogue applied to substances that have the property of removing accumulations of water or serum.

hypnotic drugs or substances that induce sleep.

irritant a general term encompassing any agent that causes irritation of a tissue.

laxative a substance that is taken to evacuate the bowel or soften stools.

mydriatic a compound that cause dilation of the pupil.

nervine a name given to drugs that are used to restore the nerves to their natural state.

narcotic a drug that leads to a stupor and complete loss of awareness.

nutritive compounds that are nourishing to the body.

pectoral applied to drugs that are a remedy in treating chest and lung complaints.

purgative the name given to drugs or other measures that produce evacuation of the bowels. This has normally a more severe effect than aperients or laxatives.

refrigerant a substance that relieves thirst and produces a feeling of coolness.

resolvent a substance that is applied to swellings to reduce them in size.

rubefacient a compound that causes the skin to redden and peel off. Causes blisters and inflammation.

sedative a drug that lessens tension, anxiety and soothes over-excitement of the nervous system.

stimulant a drug or other agent that increases the activity of an organ
or system within the body.

stomachic name given to drugs that treat stomach disorders.

styptic applications that check bleeding by blood vessel contraction or by causing rapid blood clotting.

sudorific a drug or agent that produces copious perspiration.

taenicide drugs that are used to expel tapeworms from the body.

tonic substances that are traditionally thought to give strength and vigour to the body and that are said to produce a feeling of wellbeing.

vermifuge a substance that kills, or expels, worms from the intestines.

vulnerary a drug that is said to be good at healing wounds.

Examples of herbs

Aconite *Aconitum napellus. Common /lame:* Monkshood, blue rocket, friar's cap, wolfsbane.

Occurrence: indigenous to mountain slopes in the Alps and Pyrenees. Introduced into England very early, before 900 AD.

Parts used: the leaves used fresh and the root when dried. It contains alkaloidal material-aconitine, benzaconine and aconine amongst other compounds.

Medicinal uses: the plant is poisonous and should not be used except under medical advice. It is an anodyne, diaphoretic, febrifuge and sedative. Used for reducing fever and inflammation in the treatment of catarrh, tonsillitis and croup. It may be used in controlling heart spasm.

Administered as: tincture, liniment and occasionally as hypodermic injection.

Anemone wood *Anemone nemorosa. Common name:* Crowfoot, windflower, smell fox.

Occurrence: found in woods and thickets across Great Britain.

Parts used: the root, leaves and juice.

Medicinal uses: this species of plant is much less widely used than it has been previously. It used to be good for leprosy, lethargy, eye inflammation and headaches. An ointment made of the leaves is said to be effective in cleansing malignant ulcers.

Administered as: decoction, fresh leaves and root, ointment.

Anemone pulsatilla *Anemone pulsatilla. Common name:* Pasque flower, meadow anemone, wind flower

Occurrence: found locally in chalk downs and limestone areas.

Parts used: the whole herb. It produces oil of anemone upon distillation with water.

Medicinal uses: nervi ne, antispasmodic, alterative and diaphoretic. It is beneficial in disorders of mucous membranes and of the respiratory and digestive passages. Can be used to treat asthma, whooping cough and bronchitis.

Administered as: fluid extract.

Balm *Melissa officinalis. Common name:* Sweet balm, lemon balm, honey plant, cure-all.

Occurrence: a common garden plant in Great Britain that was naturalized into southern England at a very early period.

Parts used: the herb.

Medicinal uses: as a carminative, diaphoretic, or febrifuge. It can be made into a cooling tea for fever patients and balm is often used in combination with other herbs to treat colds and fever.
Administered as: an infusion.

Belladonna Atropa belladonna. Common name: Deadly nightshade, devil's cherries, dwale, black cherry, devil's herb, great morel.

Occurrence: native to central and southern Europe but commonly grows in England.

Parts used: the roots and leaves. The root contains several alkaloid compounds including hyoscyamine, atropine and belladonnine. The same alkaloids are present in the leaves but the amount of each compound varies according to plant type and methods of storing and drying leaves.
Medicinal uses: as a narcotic, diuretic, sedative, mydriatic, antispasmodic. The drug is used as an anodyne in febrile conditions, night sweats and coughs. It is valuable in treating eye diseases and is used as a pain-relieving lotion to treat neuralgia, gout, rheumatism and sciatica. Belladonna is an extremely poisonous plant and should always be used under

medical supervision. Cases of accidental poisoning and death are well known. Despite this, it is a valuable drug used to treat a wide range of disease.

Administered as: a liquid extract that is used to produce alcoholic extracts, plasters, liniment, suppositories, tincture and ointment.

Broom Cytisus scoparius. Common name: Broom tops, Irish tops, basam, bizzom, browne, brum, bream, green broom.

Occurrence: indigenous to England and commonly found on heathland throughout Great Britain, Europe and northern Asia.

Parts used: the young herbaceous tops that contain sparteine and scoparin as the active components.

Medicinal uses: diuretic and cathartic. The broom tops may be used as a decoction or infusion to aid dropsy, while if the tops are pressed and treated broom juice is obtained. This fluid extract is generally used in combination with other diuretic compounds. An infusion of broom, agrimony and dandelion root is excellent in remedying bladder, kidney and liver trouble. Cytisus should be used carefully as the sparteine has a strong effect on the heart and, depending upon dose, can cause weakness of the heart similar to that caused by hemlock (Conium maculatum). Death can occur in extreme cases if the respiratory organ's activity is impaired.

Administered as: fluid extract and infusion.

Chamomile *Anthemis nobilis. Common name:* Roman chamomile, double chamomile, manzanilla (Spanish), may then (Saxon),

Occurrence: a low-growing plant found wild in the British Isles.
Parts used: the flowers and herb. The active principles therein are a volatile oil, anthemic acid, tannic acid and a glucoside.

Medicinal uses: tonic, stomachic, anodyne and antispasmodic. An infusion of chamomile tea was once thought to be a remedy for hysterical and nervous afflictions in women, as well as an emmenagogue. It has a powerful soothing and sedative effect that is harmless. A tincture is used to cure diarrhoea in children and it is used with purgatives to prevent griping, and as a tonic it helps dropsy. Externally, it can be applied alone or with other herbs as a poultice to relieve pain, swellings, inflammation and neuralgia. Its strong antiseptic properties make it invaluable for reducing swelling of the face due to abscess or injury. As a lotion, the flowers are good for resolving toothache and earache. The herb itself is an ingredient in herb beers. The use of chamomile can be dated back to ancient Egyptian times when they dedicated the plant to the sun because of its extensive healing properties.

Administered as: decoction, infusion, fluid extract and essential oil.

Clover, Red
Trifolium pratense. Common name: Trefoil, purple clover.

Occurrence: widely distributed in Britain and Europe.

Parts used: the flowers.

Medicinal uses: alterative, sedative, antispasmodic. The fluid extract or infusion are excellent in treating bronchial and whooping coughs. External application of the herb in a poultice has been used on cancerous growths.

Administered as: fluid extract and infusion.

Coltsfoot

Tussilago farfara. Common name: Coughwort, hall foot, horsehoof, ass's foot, foals-wort, fieldhove, bullsfoot, donnhove.

Occurrence: commonly found wild on waste ground and riverbanks in Great Britain.

Parts used: the leaves, flowers and root.

Medicinal uses: demulcent, expectorant and tonic. Coltsfoot is one of the most popular cough remedies and is generally taken in conjunction with horehound, marshmallow or ground ivy. It has been called 'Nature's best herb for the lungs' and it was recommended that the leaves be smoked to relieve a cough. Today, it forms the basis of British herb tobacco along with bogbean, eyebright, wood betony, rosemary, thyme, lavender and chamomile, which is said to relieve asthma, catarrh, bronchitis and lung troubles.

Administered as: syrup or smoked when dried.

Comfrey
Symphytum officinale. Common name: Common comfrey, knitbone, knitback, bruisewort, slippery root, gum plant, con solid a, ass ear, blackwort.

Occurrence: a native of Europe and temperate Asia but is common throughout England by rivers and ditches.

Parts used: the root and leaves. The roots contain a large quantity of mucilage, choline and allantoin.

Medicinal uses: demulcent, mildly astringent, expectorant and vulnerary. It is frequently used in pulmonary complaints, to soothe intestinal trouble and is a gentle remedy for diarrhoea and dysentery. A strong decoction or tea is administered in cases of internal haemorrhage whether it is the lungs, stomach, bowels or haemorrhoids. Externally, the leaves have been used as a poultice to promote healing of severe cuts, ulcers and abscesses and to reduce swelling, sprains and bruises. Allantoin is known to reduce swelling round damaged or fractured bones, thus allowing healing to occur faster and more thoroughly.

Administered as: a decoction, poultice and liquid extract.

Dandelion
Taraxacum officinale. Common name: Priest's crown, swine's snout.

Occurrence: widely found across the northern temperate zone in pastures, meadows and waste ground.

Parts used: the root and leaves. The main constituents of the root are taraxacin, a bitter substance, and taraxacerin, an acid resin, along with the sugar inulin.

Medicinal uses: diuretic, tonic and slightly aperient. It acts as a general body stimulant, but chiefly acts on the liver and kidneys. Dandelion is used as a bitter tonic in atonic dyspepsia as a mild laxative and to promote increased appetite and digestion. The herb is best used in combination with other herbs and is used in many patent medicines. Roasted dandelion root is also used as a coffee substitute and helps ease dyspepsia, gout and rheumatism.

Administered as: fluid extract, decoction, infusion, tincture, solid extract and juice.

Elder
Sambucus nigra. Common name: black elder, common elder, European elder, pipe tree, bore tree, bour tree.

Occurrence: frequently seen in Europe and Great Britain.

Parts used: the bark, leaves, flowers and berries.

Medicinal uses: the bark is a strong purgative and in large doses is emetic. It has been used successfully in epilepsy, and a tincture of the young bark relieves asthmatic symptoms and croup in children.

A tea made from elder roots was highly effective against dropsy. The leaves are used both fresh and dried and contain the alkaloid sambucine, a glucoside called sambunigrin, as well as hydrogenic acid, cane sugar and potassium nitrate amongst other compounds. The leaves are used in preparation of green elder ointment, which is used domestically for bruises, haemorrhoids, sprains, chilblains and applied to wounds. Elder leaves have the same purgative effects as the bark (but produce more nausea) and have expectorant, diaphoretic and diuretic actions.

The elder flowers are either distilled into elderflower water or dried. The water is used in eye and skin lotions as it is mildly astringent and a gentle stimulant. When infused, the dried flowers
make elderflower tea, which is gently laxative, aperient and diaphoretic. It is an old-fashioned remedy for colds and influenza when taken hot, before bed. The tea is also recommended
to be drunk before breakfast as a blood purifier. Elder flowers would also be made into a lotion or poultice for use on inflamed areas and into an ointment that was good on wounds, scalds and burns. The ointment was used on the battlefields in World War I and at home for chapped hands and chilblains.

Administered as: an infusion, tincture, ointment, syrup, lotion, distilled water, poultice and dried powder.

Evening primrose
Oenothera biennis. Common name: Tree primrose, sun drop.

Occurrence: native to North America but has been naturalized to British and European gardens.

Parts used: the bark and leaves.

Medicinal uses: astringent, sedative. The drug from this herb is not extensively used but has been of benefit in treating gastrointestinal disorders, dyspepsia, liver torpor and in female problems in association with pelvic illness. It has also been successfully used in whooping cough and spasmodic asthma.

Administered as.: liquid extract.

Fennel
Foeniculum vulgare. Common name: Hinojo, fenkel, sweet fennel, wild fennel.

Occurrence: found wild in most areas of temperate Europe and generally considered indigenous to the shores of the Mediterranean.
It is cultivated for medicinal benefit in France, Russia, India and Persia.

Parts used: the seeds, leaves and roots. The roots are rarely used in herbal medicine today. The essential oil is separated by distillation with water. Fennel oil varies in quality and composition dependent upon where, and under what conditions, the fennel was grown.

Medicinal uses: aromatic, stimulant, carminative and stomachic. The herb is principally used with purgatives to allay their tendency to griping, and the seeds form an ingredient of the compound liquorice powder. Fennel water also acts in a similar manner to dill water in correcting infant flatulence.

Administered as: fluid extract, distilled water, essential oil.

Foxglove

Digitalis purpurea. Common name: Witch's gloves, dead men's bells, fairy's glove, gloves of Our Lady, bloody fingers, Virgin's glove, fairy caps, folk's glove, fairy thimbles, fair women's plant.

Occurrence: indigenous and widely distributed throughout Great Britain and Europe.
Parts used: the leaves, which contain four important glucosidesdigitoxin, digitalin, digitalein and digitonin-of which the first three listed are cardiac stimulants.

Medicinal uses: cardiac tonic, sedative, diuretic. Administering digitalis increases the activity of all forms of muscle tissue, particularly the heart and arterioles. It causes a very high rise in blood pressure and the pulse is slowed and becomes regular. Digitalis causes the heart to contract in size, allowing increased blood flow and nutrient delivery to the organ. It also acts on the kidneys and is a good remedy for dropsy, particularly when it is connected with cardiac problems. The drug has benefits in treating internal haemorrhage, epilepsy, inflammatory diseases and delirium tremens. Digitalis has a cumulative action whereby it is liable to accumulate in the body and then have poisonous effects. It should only be used under medical advice. Digitalis is an excellent antidote in aconite poisoning when given as a hypodermic injection.

Administered as: tincture, infusion, powdered leaves, injection.

Golden rod

Solidago virgaurea. Common name: Verge d'or, solidago, goldruthe, woundwort, Aaron's Rod.

Occurrence: this is a plant normally found wild in woods in Great Britain, Europe, Central Asia and North America but it is also a common garden plant.

Parts used: the leaves contain tannin, with some bitter and astringent chemicals that are unknown.

Medicinal uses: aromatic, stimulant, carminative. This herb is astringent and diuretic and is highly effective in curing gravel and urinary stones. It aids weak digestion, stops sickness and is very good against diphtheria. As a warm infusion it is a good diaphoretic drug and is used as such to help painful menstruation and amenorrhoea (absence or stopping of menstrual periods).

Administered as: fluid extract, infusion, spray.

Hemlock
Conium maculatum. Common name: Herb bennet, spotted conebane, musquash root, beaver poison, poison hemlock, poison parsley, spotted hemlock, vex, vecksies.

Occurrence: common in hedges, meadows, waste ground and stream banks throughout Europe and is also found in temperate Asia and north Africa.

Parts used: the leaves, fruits and seeds. The most important constituent of hemlock leaves is the alkaloid coniine, which is poisonous, with a disagreeable odour. Other alkaloids in the plant include methyl-coniine, conhydrine, pseudoconhydrine, ethyl piperidine.

Medicinal uses: sedative, antispasmodic, anodyne. The drug acts on the centres of motion and causes paralysis and so it is used to remedy nervous motor excitability, e.g. teething, cramp and muscle spasms of the larynx and gullet. When inhaled, hemlock is said to be good in relieving coughs, bronchitis, whooping cough and asthma. The method of action of *Conium* means it is directly antagonistic to the effects of strychnine, from nux vomica *(Strychnos nux-vomica),* and it is used as an antidote to strychnine poisoning and similar poisons. Hemlock has to be administered with care as narcotic poisoning may result from internal application and overdoses induce paralysis, with loss of speech and depression of respiratory function leading to death. Antidotes to hemlock poisoning are tannic acid, stimulants, e.g. coffee, mustard and castor oil.

Administered as: powdered leaves, fluid extract, tincture, expressed juice of the leaves and solid extract.

Honeysuckle
Lonicera caprifolium. Common name: Dutch honeysuckle, goat's leaf, perfoliate honeysuckle.

Occurrence: it grows freely in Europe, Great Britain and through the northern temperate zone.
Parts used: the dried flowers and leaves.

Medicinal uses: expectorant, laxative. A syrup made of the flowers is used for respiratory diseases and asthma. A decoction of the leaves is laxative and is also good against diseases of the liver and spleen, and in gargles.

Administered as: syrup, decoction.

Juniper
Juniperus communis.

Occurrence: a common shrub native to Great Britain and widely distributed through many parts of the world.

Parts used: the berry and leaves.

Medicinal uses: the oil of juniper obtained from the ripe berries is stomachic, diuretic and carminative and is used to treat indigestion and flatulence as well as kidney and bladder diseases. The main use of juniper is in dropsy, and aiding other diuretic herbs to ease the disease.

Administered as: essential oil from berries, essential oil from wood, fluid extract, liquid extract, solid extract.

Larch
Pinus larix. Common name: Larix europaea, Abies larix, Larix decidua, Laricus cortex, European larch, Venice turpentine.

Occurrence: indigenous to hilly regions of central Europe, but was introduced into Great Britain in 1639.

Parts used: the inner bark, which contains tannic acid, larixinic acid and turpentine.

Medicinal uses: stimulant, diuretic, astringent, balsamic and expectorant. It is very useful as an external application for eczema and psoriasis. However, it is mainly used as a stimulant expectorant in chronic bronchitis and for internal haemorrhage and cystitis. Larch turpentine has also been suggested as an antidote in cyanide or opium poisoning and has been used as a hospital disinfectant.

Administered as: fluid extract or syrup.

Liquorice
Glycyrrhiza glabra. Common name: Licorice,lycorys, Liquiriha officinalis.
Occurrence: a shrub native to southeast Europe and southwest Asia.

Parts used: the root. The chief compound in the root is glychrrhizin along with sugar, starch, gum, tannin and resin.

Medicinal uses: demulcent, pectoral, emollient. A very popular and well-known remedy for coughs, consumption and chest complaints. Liquorice extract is included in cough lozenges and pastilles, with sedatives and expectorants. An infusion of bruised root and flax (linseed) is good for irritable coughs, sore throats and laryngitis. Liquorice is used to a greater extent as a medicine in China and other eastern countries. The herb is used by brewers to give colour to porter and stout and is employed in the manufacture of chewing or smoking tobacco.

Administered as: powdered root, fluid extract, infusion, solid extract.

Meadowsweet
Spiraea ulmaria. Common name: Meadsweet, dolloff, queen of the meadow, bridewort, lady of the meadow. *Occurrence:* a common wild plant in the British Isles, found growing in meadows or woods.

Parts used: the herb.

Medicinal uses: aromatic, astringent, diuretic, alterative. This herb is good against diarrhoea, stomach complaints and blood disorders. It is highly recommended for children's diarrhoea and dropsy and was used as a decoction in wine to reduce fevers. Meadowsweet makes a pleasant everyday drink when infused and sweetened with honey. It is also included in many herb beers.

Administered as: infusion, decoction.

Nettle
Urtica dioica, Urtica urens. Common name: Common nettle, stinging nettle.

Occurrence: widely distributed throughout temperate Europe and Asia, Japan, South Africa and Australia.

Parts used: the whole herb, which contains formic acid, mucilage, mineral salts, ammonia and carbonic acid.

Medicinal uses: astringent, stimulating, diuretic, tonic. The herb is anti-asthmatic and the juice of the nettle will relieve bronchial and asthmatic troubles, as will the dried leaves when burnt and inhaled. The seeds are taken as an infusion or in wine to ease consumption or ague. Nettles are used widely as a food source and are made into puddings, tea, beer, juice and used as a vegetable. A hair tonic or lotion can also be made from the herb. In the Highlands of Scotland, they were chopped, added to egg white and applied to the temples as a cure for insomnia.

Administered as: expressed juice, infusion, decoction, seeds, dried herb, dietary item.

Peppermint *Mentha piperita. Common name:* Brandy mint, curled mint, balm mint.

Occurrence: found across Europe, was introduced into Britain and grows widely in damp places and waste ground.

Parts used: the herb and distilled oil. The plant contains peppermint oil, which is composed of menthol, menthyl acetate and isovalerate, menthone, cineol. pinene and limonene. The medicinal qualities are found in the alcoholic chemicals.

Medicinal uses: stimulant, antispasmodic, carminative, stomachic, oil of peppermint is extensively used in both medicine and commerce. It is good in dyspepsia, flatulence, colic and abdominal cramps. The oil allays sickness and nausea, is used for chorea and diarrhoea but is normally used with other medicines to disguise unpalatable tastes and effects. Peppermint water is in most general use and is used to raise body temperature and induce perspiration. Peppermint tea can help ward off colds and influenza at an early stage, can calm heart palpitations and is used to reduce the appetite.

Administered as: infusion, distilled water, spirit, essential oil and fluid extract.

Primrose *Primula vulgaris.*

Occurrence: a common wild flower found in woods, hedgerows and pastures throughout Great Britain.

Parts used: the root and whole herb. Both parts of the plant contain a fragrant oil called primulin and the active principle saponin.

Medicinal uses: astringent, antispasmodic, vermifuge, emetic. It was formerly considered to be an important remedy in muscular rheumatism, paralysis and gout. A tincture of the whole plant has sedative effects and is used successfully in extreme sensitivity, restlessness and insomnia. Nervous headaches can be eased by treatment with an infusion of the root, while the powdered dry root serves as an emetic. An infusion of Primrose flowers is excellent in nervous headaches and an ointment can be made out of the leaves to heal and salve wounds and cuts.

Administered as: infusion, tincture, powdered root and ointment.

Ragwort
Senecio jacobaea. Common name: St James's wort, stinking nanny, staggerwort, ragweed, dog standard, cankerwort, stammerwort, fireweed.

Occurrence: an abundant wild plant, widely distributed over Great Britain, Europe, Siberia and northwest India.

Parts used: the herb.
Medicinal uses: diaphoretic, detergent, emollient, cooling, astringent. The leaves were used as emollient poultices, while the expressed juice of the herb was utilized as a wash in burns, eye inflammation, sores and cancerous ulcers. It has been

successful in relieving rheumatism, sciatica, gout and in reducing inflammation and swelling of joints when applied as a poultice. Ragwort makes a good gargle for ulcerated throats and mouths and a decoction of its root is said to help internal bruising and wounds. The herb was previously thought to be able to prevent infection. This plant is poisonous to cattle and should be removed from their pastures. The alkaloids in the ragwort have cumulative effects in the cattle and low doses of the chemical eaten over a period of time can built up to a critical level, where the cattle show obvious symptoms and then die. It is uncertain if sheep are also susceptible to this chemical.

Administered as: poultice, infusion and decoction .

Rosemary
Rosmarinus officinalis. Common name: Polar plant, compass-weed, compass plant, romero, *Rosmarinus coronarium.*

Occurrence: native to the dry hills of the Mediterranean, from Spain westward to Turkey. A common garden plant in Britain, having been cultivated prior to the Norman Conquest.

Parts used: the herb and root. Oil of rosemary is distilled from the plant tops and used medicinally. Rosemary contains tannic acid, a bitter principle, resin and a volatile oil.

Medicinal uses: tonic, astringent, diaphoretic, stimulant. The essential oil is also stomachic, nervi ne and carminative and cures many types of headache. It is mainly applied externally as a hair lotion that is said to prevent baldness and the formation of dandruff. The oil is used externally as a rubefacient and is added to liniments for fragrance and stimulant properties. Rosemary tea can remove headache, colic, colds and nervous diseases and may also lift nervous depression.

Administered as: infusion, essential oil and lotion.

Sorrel

Rumex acetosa. Common name: Garden sorrel, green sauce, sour grabs, sour suds, cuckoo sorrow, cuckoo's meate, gowke-meat.

Occurrence: indigenous to Britain and found in moist meadows throughout Europe.

Parts used: the leaves, dried and fresh.

Medicinal uses: refrigerant, diuretic, antiscorbutic. Sorrel is given as a cooling drink in all febrile conditions and can help correct scrofulous deposits. Its astringent qualities meant it was formerly used to stop haemorrhages and was applied as a poultice on cutaneous tumours. Sorrel juice and vinegar are said to cure ringworm, while a decoction was made to cure jaundice, ulcerated bowel, and gravel and stone in the kidneys.

Administered as: expressed juice, decoction, poultice and dried leaves.

Tansy

Tanacetum vulgare. Common name: Buttons.
Occurrence: a hardy perennial plant, commonly seen on waste ground all over Europe and Great Britain.

Parts used: the herb. It contains the chemicals tanacetin, tannic acid, a volatile oil, thujone, sugar and a colouring matter among others.

Medicinal uses: anthelmintic, tonic, emmenagogue, stimulant. Tansy is largely used for expelling worms from children. The herb is also used for slight fevers, for allaying spasms and as a nervine drug. In large doses, the herb is violently irritant and induces venous congestion of the abdominal organs. In Scotland, an infusion was administered to cure gout. Tansy essential oil, when given in small doses, has helped in epilepsy and has also been used externally to help some eruptive diseases of the skin. Bruised fresh leaves can reduce swelling and relieve sprains, as can a hot infusion used as a poultice.

Administered as: essential oil, infusion, poultice, fresh leaves, solid extract.

Thyme
Thymus vulgaris. Common name: Garden or common thyme, tomillo.

Occurrence: cultivated in temperate countries in northern Europe.

Parts used: the herb. Thyme gives rise to oil of thyme after distillation of the fresh leaves. This oil contains the phenols, thymol and carvacrol, as well as cymene, pinene and borneol.

Medicinal uses: antiseptic, antispasmodic, tonic, carminative. The fresh herb, in syrup, forms a safe cure for whooping cough, as is an infusion of the dried herb. The infusion or tea is beneficial for catarrh, sore throat, wind spasms, colic and in allaying fevers and colds. Thyme is generally used in conjunction with other remedies in herbal medicine.

Administered as: fluid extract, essential oil and infusion.

Valerian
Valeriana officinalis. Common name: all-heal, great wild valerian, amantilla, setwall, sete-wale, capon's tail.

Occurrence: found throughout Europe and northern Asia. It is common in England in marshy thickets, riverbanks and ditches.

Parts used: the root, which contains a volatile oil, two alkaloids called chatarine and Valerianine as well as several unidentified compounds.

Medicinal uses: powerful nervine, stimulant, carminative anodyne and antispasmodic herb. It may be given in all cases of nervous debility and irritation as it is not narcotic. The expressed juice of the fresh root has been used as a narcotic in insomnia and as an anticonvulsant in epilepsy. The oil of valerian is of use against cholera and in strengthening the eyesight. A herbal compound containing valerian was given to civilians during the Second World War, to reduce the effects of stress caused by repeated air raids and to minimize damage to health.

Administered as: fluid extract, tincture, essential oil, expressed juice.

Witch hazel
Hamamelis virginiana. Common name: Spotted alder, winterbloom, snapping hazelnut.
Occurrence: native to the United States of America and Canada.

Parts used: the dried bark, both fresh and dried leaves. The leaves contain tannic and gallic acids, volatile oil and an unknown bitter principle. The bark contains tannin, gallic acid, a physterol, resin, fat and other bitter and odorous bodies.

Medicinal uses: astringent, tonic, sedative. Valuable in stopping internal and external haemorrhages and in treating piles. Mainly used for bruises, swelling, inflammation and tumours as a poultice.
It may also be utilized for diarrhoea, dysentery and mucous discharges. A decoction is used against tuberculosis, gonorrhoea, menorrhagia and the debilitated state resulting from abortion. Tea made from the bark or leaves aids bleeding of the stomach, bowel complaints and may be given as an injection for bleeding piles. Witch hazel is used to treat varicose veins as a moist poultice, as an extract to ease burns, scalds and

insect and mosquito bites, and to help inflammation of the eyelids.

Administered as: liquid extract, injection, tincture, lotion, ointment, suppositories, poultice, infusion and decoction.

Homoeopathy

Introduction

The aim of homoeopathy is to cure an illness or disorder by treating the whole person rather than merely concentrating on a set of symptoms. Hence, in homoeopathy the approach is holistic, and the overall state of health of the patient, especially his or her emotional and psychological wellbeing, is regarded as being very significant. A homoeopath notes the symptoms that the person wishes to have cured, but also takes time to discover other signs or indications of disorder that the patient may regard as being less important. The reasoning behind this is that illness is a sign of disorder or imbalance within the body. It is believed that the whole 'make-up' of a person determines, to a great extent, the type of disorders to which that individual is prone and the symptoms likely to occur. A homoeopathic remedy must be suitable both for the symptoms and the characteristics and temperament of the patient. Hence, two patients with the same illness may be offered different remedies according to their individual natures. One remedy may also be used to treat different groups of symptoms or ailments.

Homoeopathic remedies are based on the concept that 'like cures like', an ancient philosophy that can be traced back to the 5th century BC when it was formulated by Hippocrates.In the early 1800s, this idea awakened the interest of a German doctor, Samuel Hahnemann, who believed that the medical practices at that time were too harsh and tended to hinder rather than aid healing. Hahnemann observed that a treatment for malaria, based on an extract of cinchona bark (quinine), actually produced symptoms of this disease when taken in a small dose by a healthy person. Further extensive studies convinced him that the production of symptoms was the body's way of combating illness. Hence, to give a minute dose of a substance that stimulated the symptoms of an illness in a healthy person, could be used to fight that illness in someone who was sick. Hahnemann conducted numerous trials (called 'provings') giving minute doses of substances to healthy people and recording the symptoms produced. Eventually, these very dilute remedies were given to people with illnesses, often with very encouraging results.

Modern homoeopathy is based on the work of Hahnemann, and the medicines derived from plant, mineral and animal sources are used in extremely dilute amounts. Indeed it is believed that the curative properties are enhanced by each dilution because impurities that might cause unwanted side effects are lost. Substances used in homoeopathy are first soaked in alcohol to extract their essential ingredients. This initial solution, called the 'mother tincture' is diluted successively either by factors often (called the 'decimal scale' and designated X), or 100 (the 'centesimal scale' and designated C). Each dilution is shaken vigorously before further ones are made and this is thought to make the properties more powerful by adding energy at each stage, while impurities are removed. The thorough shakings of each dilution are said to energize or 'potentiate' the medicine. The remedies are made into tablets or may be used in the form of ointment, solutions, powders, suppositories, etc. High potency (i.e. more dilute) remedies are used for severe symptoms and lower potency (less dilute) for milder ones.

The homoeopathic view is that during the process of healing, symptoms are redirected from more important to less important body systems. It is also held that healing is from innermost to outermost parts of the body and that more recent symptoms disappear first, this being known as the 'law of direction of cure'. Occasionally, symptoms may worsen initially when a homoeopathic remedy is taken, but this is usually short-lived and is known as a 'healing crisis.' It is taken to indicate a change and that improvement is likely to follow. Usually, with a homoeopathic remedy,' an improvement is noticed fairly quickly although this depends upon the nature of the ailment, health, age and wellbeing of the patient and potency of the remedy. A first homoeopathic consultation is likely to last about I hour so that the specialist can obtain a full picture of the patient's medical history and personal circumstances. On the basis of this information, the homoeopathic doctor decides on an appropriate remedy and potency (which is usually 6C). Subsequent consultations are generally shorter and full advice is given on how to store and take the medicine. It is widely accepted that homoeopathic remedies are very safe and non-addictive but they are covered by the legal requirements governing all medicines and should be obtained from a recognized source.

Potency table for homoeopathic medicines

The centesimal scale
1C = 1/100 ($1/100^1$) of mother tincture
2C = 1/10 000 ($1/100^2$) of mother tincture
3C = 1/1 000 000 ($1/100^3$) of mother tincture
6C = 1/1 000 000 000 000 ($1/100^6$) of mother tincture

The decimal scale
1X = 1/10 ($1/10^1$) of mother tincture
2X = 1/100 ($1/10^2$) of mother tincture
6X = 1/1 000 000 ($1/10^6$) of mother tincture

The development of homoeopathy

The Greek physician, Hippocrates, who lived several hundred years before the birth of Christ (460-370 BC), is regarded as the founding father of all medicine. The Hippocratic Oath taken by newly qualified doctors in orthodox medicine binds them to an ethical code of medical practice in honour of Hippocrates. Hippocrates believed that disease resulted from natural elements in the world
in which people lived. This contrasted with the view that held sway for centuries that disease was some form of punishment

from the gods or God. He believed that it was essential to observe and take account of the course and progress of a disease in each individual, and that any cure should encourage that person's own innate healing power. Hippocrates embraced the idea of 'like being able to cure like' and had many remedies that were based on this principle. Hence in his practice and study of medicine he laid the foundations of the homoeopathic approach although this was not to be appreciated and developed for many centuries.

During the period of Roman civilization a greater knowledge and insight into the nature of the human body was developed. Many herbs and plants were used for healing by people throughout the world, and much knowledge was gained and handed down from generation to generation. However, the belief persisted that diseases were caused by supernatural or divine forces. It was not until the early 1500s that a Swiss doctor, Paracelsus (1493-1541) put forward the view that disease resulted from external environmental forces. He also believed that plants and natural substances held the key to healing and embraced the 'like can cure like' principle. One of his ideas, known as the Doctrine of Signatures, was that the appearance of a plant, or the substances it contained, gave an idea of the disorders it could cure.

In the succeeding centuries, increased knowledge was gained about the healing properties of plants and the way the human body worked. In spite of this, the methods of medical practice were extremely harsh and there is no doubt that many people suffered needlessly and died due to the treatment they received. It was against this background that Samuel Hahnemann, (1755-1843) the founding father of modern homoeopathy, began his work as a doctor in the late 1700s. In his early writings, Hahnemann criticized the severe practices of medicine and advocated a healthy diet, clean living conditions and high standards of hygiene as a means of improving health and warding off disease. In 1790, he became interested in quinine, extracted from the bark of the cinchona tree, which was known to be an effective treatment for malaria. He tested the substance first on himself, and later on friends and close family members and recorded the results, and these early experiments were called 'provings'. The results led him to conduct many further investigations and provings of other natural substances, during the course of which he rediscovered and established the principle of like being able to cure like.

By 1812, the principle and practice of homoeopathy, based on the work of Hahnemann, had become established and many other doctors adopted the homoeopathic approach. Hahnemann himself become a teacher in homoeopathy at the University of Leipzig and published many important writings-the results of his years of research. He continued to practice, teach and conduct research throughout his life, especially in producing more dilute remedies that were succussed or shaken at each stage and were found to be more potent. Although his work was not without its detractors, Hahnemann had attracted a considerable following by the 1830s. In 1831, there was a widespread cholera epidemic in central Europe for which Hahnemann recommended treatment with camphor. Many people were cured, including Dr Frederick Quin, (1799-1878), a medical practitioner at that time. He went on to establish the first homoeopathic hospital in London in 1849. A later resurgence of cholera in Britain enabled the effectiveness of camphor to be established beyond doubt, as the numbers of people cured at the homoeopathic hospital were far greater than those treated at other hospitals.

In the United States of America, homoeopathy became firmly established in the early part of the 19th century and there were several eminent practitioners who further enhanced knowledge and practice. These included Dr Constantine Hering (1800-1880), who formulated the Laws of Cure, explaining how symptoms affect organ systems and move from one part of the body to another as a cure occurs. Dr James Tyler Kent (1849-1916) introduced the idea of constitutional types, which is now the basis of classical homoeopathy, and advocated the use of high potency remedies.

In the later years of the 19th century, a fundamental split occurred in the practice of homoeopathy, which was brought about by Dr Richard Hughes (1836--1902), who worked in London and Brighton. He insisted that physical symptoms and the nature of the disease itself were the important factors rather than the holistic approach, based on the make-up of the whole individual person. Hughes rejected the concept of constitutional types and advocated the use of low-potency remedies. Although he worked as a homoeopath, his approach was to attempt to make homoeopathy more scientific and to bring it closer to the practices of conventional medicine. Some other homoeopathic doctors followed the approach of Hughes, and the split led to a collapse in faith in the whole practice of homoeopathy during the early part of the century. However, as the century advanced, homoeopathy regained its following and respect. Conventional medicine and homoeopathy have continued to advance, and there is now a greater sympathy and understanding between the practitioners in both these important disciplines.

Among homoeopathic remedies there are a small number of fundamental, regularly used compounds that are effective in treating many complaints. These are described below.

Basic remedies

Argenticum nitricum
Argent nit; silver nitrate, devil's stone, lunar caustic, hell stone. Silver nitrate is obtained from the mineral acanthite, which is a natural ore of silver. White silver nitrate crystals are derived from a chemical solution of the mineral ore, and these are used

to make the homoeopathic remedy. Silver nitrate is poisonous in large doses and has antiseptic and caustic properties. In the past it was used to clean out wounds and prevent infection. In homoeopathy, it is used to treat states of great anxiety, panic, fear or apprehension about a forthcoming event, e.g. taking an examination, having to perform a public role (speech-making, chairing a public meeting, acting, singing), going for an interview or any activity involving scrutiny and criticism by others. It was also used as a remedy for digestive complaints including indigestion, abdominal pain, wind, nausea and also for headache. Often, there is a longing for sweet 'comfort' or other types of food. Argent nit. may be given for laryngitis, sore throat and hoarseness, eye inflammation such as conjunctivitis and for period pains. Other types of pain, asthma and warts may benefit from argent nit.

Often, a person experiences symptoms mainly on the left side and these are worse for heat and at night. Also, they are made worse by anxiety and overwork, emotional tension and resting on the left side. Pains are made worse with talking and movement. Symptoms improve in cold or cool fresh air and are relieved by belching. Pains are helped by applying pressure to the painful part. People suitable for argent nit. are quick-witted and rapid in thought and action. They may appear outgoing and happy but are a prey to worry, anxiety and ungrounded fears that make them tense. All the emotions are quick to surface and argent nit. people are able to put on an impressive performance. They enjoy a wide variety of foods, particularly salty and sweet things, although these may upset the digestion. They have a fear of heights, crowds, of being burgled, of failure, and arriving late for an appointment. They also have a fear of serious illness, dying and madness. Argent nit. people are generally slim and full of restless energy and tension. They may have deeply etched features and lines on the skin that make them appear older than their actual age.

Arsenicum album

Arsen alb; white arsenic trioxide.

This is a widely used homoeopathic remedy, the source being white arsenic trioxide derived from arsenopyrite, a metallic mineral ore of arsenic. Arsenic has been known for centuries as a poison and was once used as a treatment for syphilis. White arsenic trioxide used to be given to improve muscles and skin in animals such as horses. It is used to treat acute conditions of the digestive system and chest and mental symptoms of anxiety and fear. Hence it is a remedy for diarrhoea and vomiting caused by eating the wrong kinds of food, or food poisoning or over-indulgence in alcohol. Also, for dehydration in children following gas troenteritis or feverish illness. It is a remedy for asthma and breathing difficulty, mouth ulcers, carbuncle (a collection of boils), dry, cracked lips, burning skin, inflamed, watering stinging eyes and psoriasis. Also, for sciatica, shingles, sore throat and painful swallowing, candidiasis (fungal infection) of the mouth and motion sickness. There may be oedema (retention of fluid) showing as a puffiness around the ankles.

An ill person who benefits from arsen alb. experiences burning pains but also feels cold. The skin may be either hot or cold to the touch. The symptoms are worse for cold in any form, including cold food and drink, and between midnight and 3 a.m. They are worse on the right side and if the person is near the coast. Symptoms improve with warmth (including warm drinks), gentle movement and lying down with the head raised. People suitable for arsen alb. are precise, meticulous and ambitious and loathe any form of disorder. They are always immaculately dressed and everything in their life is neat and tidy. However, they tend to have great worries, especially about their financial security and their own health and that of their family. They fear illness and dying, loss of financial and personal status, being burgled, darkness and the supernatural. Arsen alb. people have strongly held views and do not readily tolerate contrary opinions or those with a more relaxed or disordered lifestyle.

They enjoy a variety of different foods, coffee and alcoholic drinks. They are usually thin, with delicate, fine features and pale skin that may show worry lines. Their movements tend to be rapid and their manner serious and somewhat restless, although they are always polite.

Calcarea carbonica
Calc. carb; calcium carbonate.

This important homoeopathic remedy is made from powdered mother-of-pearl, the beautiful, translucent inner layer of oyster shells. Calcium is an essential mineral in the body, being especially important for the healthy development of bones and teeth. The calc. carbo remedy is used to treat a number of different disorders especially those relating to bones and teeth, but also certain skin conditions and symptoms relating to the female reproductive system. It is a remedy for weak or slow growth of bones and teeth and fractures that take a long time to heal. Also, for teething problems in children, pains in bones, teeth and joints, headaches and eye inflammations affecting the right side, and ear infections with an unpleasant-smelling discharge. Premenstrual syndrome, heavy periods and menopausal disorders are helped by calc. carb, and also chapped skin and eczema.

Calc. carbo may be used as a remedy for verruca (a type of wart) and thrush infections. People who benefit from calc. carbo are very sensitive to the cold, particularly in the hands and feet and tend to sweat profusely. They suffer from fatigue and anxiety, and body secretions (sweat and urine) smell unpleasant. Children who benefit from calc. carbo have recurrent ear, nose and throat infections, especially tonsillitis and glue ear. Symptoms are made worse by draughts and cold, damp weather and also at night. They are worse when the person first wakens in the morning and for physical exercise and sweating. In women, symptoms are worse premenstrually. They improve in warm, dry weather and are better later on in the morning and after the person has eaten breakfast.

People suitable for calc. carbo are often overweight or even obese with a pale complexion. They are shy and very sensitive, quiet in company and always worried about what other people think of them. Calc. carbo people are hard-working, conscientious and reliable and easily upset by the suffering of others. They need constant reassurance from friends and family and tend to feel that they are a failure. Usually, calc. carbo people enjoy good health but have a tendency for skeletal weakness. They enjoy a wide variety of different foods and tend to overeat, but are upset by coffee and milk. They are afraid of dying and serious illness, the supernatural, madness, being a failure and becoming poor and they tend to be claustrophobic.

Graphites

Graphite; black pencil lead

Graphite is a form of carbon that is the basis of all life. It is found in older igneous or metamorphic rocks, such as granite and marble and is mined for its industrial uses, e.g. in batteries, motors, pencil leads, cleaning and lubricating fluids. It was investigated and proved by Hahnemann after he learned that it was being used by some factory workers to heal cold sores. The powder used in homoeopathy is ground graphite and it is mainly used for skin disorders that may be caused by metabolic imbalances and stomach ulcers. It is a remedy for eczema, psoriasis, acne, rough, dry skin conditions with pustules or blisters, scarring and thickened cracked nails and cold sores. Also, for stomach ulcers due to a thinning or weakness in the lining of the stomach wall, problems caused by excessive catarrh, loss of hair and cramping pains or numbing of the feet and hands. In women it is used to treat some menstrual problems. The symptoms are worse in draughty, cold and damp conditions and for eating sweet meals or sea foods. Also, the use of steroids for skin complaints and, in women, during menstruation. Symptoms are often worse on the left side. They improve with warmth, as long as the air is fresh and it is not stuffy, when it is dark and with eating and sleep. People suitable for graphites are usually well built and may be overweight, often having dark hair. They like to eat well but lack physical fitness and sweat or flush with slight exertion. They are prone to dry, flaky skin conditions that may affect the scalp. Graphites people are usually lethargic and may be irritable, lacking in concentration for intellectual activities. They are prone to mood swings and subject to bouts of weeping, especially when listening to music. A graphites person feels that he or she is unlucky and is inclined to self-pity, often feeling fearful and timid.

Ignatia amara
Agnate; strychnos Ignatii, St Ignatius' bean
Ignatia amara is a large tree that is native to the Philippine Islands, China and the East Indies. The tree has many branches and twining stems and produces stalked white flowers. Later, seed pods are produced, each containing ten to twenty large, oval seeds, that are about one inch long and are embedded in pulp. The seeds are highly poisonous and contain strychnine, which affects the central nervous system. Similar active constituents and properties are found in *Nux vomica*. The tree is named after the founder of the Jesuits, Ignatius Loyola (1491-1556), and Spanish priests belonging to this order brought the seeds to Europe during the 1600s. The homoeopathic remedy is made from the powdered seeds and is used especially for emotional symptoms. It is used for grief, bereavement, shock and loss, particularly when a person is having difficulty coming to terms with his or her feelings and is inclined to suppress the natural responses. Accompanying symptoms include sleeplessness, anger and hysteria. Similar emotional and psychological problems are helped by this remedy, including anxiety and fear especially of appearing too forward to others, a tendency to burst into fits of crying, self-doubt, pity, blame and depression. Nervous tension headaches and digestive upsets, feverish symptoms, chills and pains in the abdomen may be helped by *Ignatia*. Some problems associated with menstruation, especially sharp pains or absence of periods, are relieved by this remedy as are conditions with changeable

symptoms. These are worse in cold weather or conditions, with emotional trauma, being touched, for smoking and drinking coffee. They improve with warmth, moving about, eating, lying on the side or area that is painful and after passing urine.

The person for whom *Ignatia* is suitable is usually female and with a tendency towards harsh, self-criticism and blame; she is usually a creative, artistic person, highly sensitive but with a tendency to suppress the emotions. She is perceptive and intelligent but inclined to be hysterical and subject to erratic mood swings. Typically, the person expects a high standard in those she loves. The person enjoys dairy products, bread and sour foods but sweets, alcoholic drinks and fruit upset her system. She is afraid of crowds, tends to be claustrophobic, and fears being burgled. Also, she is afraid of being hurt emotionally, and is very sensitive to pain. The person is usually dark-haired and of slim build with a worried expression and prone to sighing, yawning and excessive blinking.

Lachesis
Trigonocephalus lachesis; lachesis muta, venom of the bushmaster or Surukuku snake This South African snake produces a deadly venom that may
prove instantly fatal due to its effects upon the heart. The veno causes the blood to thin and flow more freely, hence increasing the likelihood of haemorrhage. Even a slight bite bleeds copiously with a risk of blood poisoning or septicaemia. The snake is a ferocious hunter and its African name, Surukuku describes the sound it makes while in pursuit of prey. The properties of the venom were investigated in the 1800s by the eminent American homoeopathic doctor, Constantine Hering , who tested and proved the remedy on himself. It is effective in treating a variety of disorders, particularly those relating to the blood circulation and where there is a risk of blood poisoning or septicaemia. It is used to treat varicose veins and problems of the circulation indicated by a bluish tinge to the skin. The remedy is useful for those suffering from a weak heart or

angina, palpitations and an irregular, fast or weak pulse. There may be symptoms of chest pain and breathing difficulty. It is of great benefit in treating uterine problems, particularly premenstrual congestion and pain that is relieved once the period starts. Also, this is an excellent remedy for menopausal symptoms; especially hot flushes, and for infections of the bladder and rectum. It is used to treat conditions and infections where symptoms are mainly on the left side, such as headache or stroke when the left side is involved. Also, as a treatment for sore throats and throat infections, tonsillitis, lung abscess, boils, ulcers, wounds that only heal slowly, vomiting due to appendicitis and digestive disorders, fevers with chills and shivering, nosebleeds and bleeding piles.

It is used to treat severe symptoms of measles and serious infections including scarlet feverand smallpox. Symptoms are made worse for touch and after sleep and by tight clothing. They are worse for hot drinks and baths, and exposure to hot sun or direct heat in any form. For women, symptoms are worse during the menopause. They improve with being out in the fresh air and drinking cold drinks and with release of normal bodily discharges. People suitable for Lachesis tend to be intelligent, creative, intense and ambitious. They have strong views about politics and world affairs and may be impatient of the views of others. They may be somewhat self-centred, possessive and jealous, which can cause problems in close relationships with others. They dislike being tied down and so may be reluctant to commit themselves to a relationship. Lachesis people have a liking for sour pickled foods, bread, rice and oysters and alcoholic drinks. They like coffee, but hot drinks and wheat-based food tends to upset them. They have a fear of water, people they do not know, being burgled and of dying or being suffocated. Lachesis people may be somewhat overweight and are sometimes red-haired and freckled. Alternatively, they may be thin and dark-haired, pale and with a lot of energy. Children tend to be somewhat jealous of others and possessive of their friends, which can lead to naughty or trying behaviour.

Lycopodium clavatum

Lycopodium; club moss, wolf's claw, vegetable sulphur, stagshorn moss, running pine

This plant is found throughout the northern hemisphere, in high moorlands, forests and mountains. The plant produces spore cases on the end of upright forked stalks, which contain the spores. These produce yellow dust or powder that is resistant to water and was once used as a coating on pills and tablets to keep them separate from one another. The powder was also used as a constituent of fireworks. It has been used medicinally for many centuries, as a remedy for digestive disorders and kidney stones in Arabian countries and in the treatment of gout. The powder and spores are collected by shaking the fresh, flowering stalks of the plant and its main use in homoeopathy is for digestive and kidney disorders. It is used to treat indigestion, heartburn, the effects of eating a large meal late at night, sickness, nausea, wind, bloatedness and constipation.

Also, in men, for kidney stones, with the production of a red-coloured urine containing a sand-like sediment and enlarged prostate gland. It is used in the treatment of some problems of male impotence and bleeding haemorrhoids or piles. Symptoms that occur on the right side are helped by *Lycopodium,* and the patient additionally tends to crave sweet, comfort foods. Nettlerash, psoriasis affecting the hands, fatigue due to illness and ME (Myalgic encephalomyelitis), some types of headache, cough and sore throat are relieved by this remedy. It is used to relieve emotional states of anxiety, fear and apprehension caused by chronic insecurity, or relating to forthcoming events such as taking an examination or appearing in public (stage fright). Also, night terrors, sleeplessness, shouting or talking in the sleep and being frightened on first waking up can all benefit from this treatment.

The symptoms are worse between 4 p.m. and 8 p.m. and in warm, stuffy rooms and with wearing clothes that are too tight. They are also worse in the early morning between 4 a.m. and 8 a.m., for eating too much and during the Spring. They improve outside in cool fresh air, after a hot meal or drink and with loosening tight clothing, with light exercise and at night. People suitable for *Lycopodium* tend to be serious, hard-working and intelligent, often in professional positions. They seem to be self-possessed and confident but are, in reality, rather insecure with a low self-opinion. They are impatient of what they perceive as being weakness and are not tolerant or sympathetic of illness. *Lycopodium* people are sociable but may keep their distance and not get involved; they may be sexually promiscuous. They have a great liking for sweet foods of all kinds and enjoy hot meals and drinks. They are easily filled but may carry on eating regardless of this and usually complain of symptoms on the right side. *Lycopodium* people are afraid of being left on their own, of failure in life, of crowds, darkness and the supernatural and tend to be claustrophobic. They are often tall, thin and pale with receding hair or hair that turns grey early in life. They may be bald, with a forehead lined with worry lines and a serious appearance. They tend to have weak muscles and are easily tired after physical exercise. They may have a tendency to unconsciously twitch the muscles of the face and to flare the nostrils.

Mercurius solubilise
Mere sol; quicksilver

The mineral cinnabar, which is found in volcanic crystalline rocks, is an important ore of mercury and is extracted for a variety of uses, including dental fillings and in thermometers. Mercury is toxic in large doses, and an affected person produces copious quantities of saliva and suffers repeated bouts of vomiting. Mercury has been used since ancient times and was once given as a remedy for syphilis. A powder of precipitate of mercury is obtained from dissolving liquid mercury in a dilute solution of nitric acid, and this is the source of the remedy used in homoeopathy. It is used as a remedy for conditions that produce copious bodily secretions that often smell unpleasant, with accompanying symptoms of heat or burning and a great sensitivity to temperature. It is used as a remedy for fevers with profuse, unpleasant sweating, bad breath, inflammation of the gums, mouth ulcers, candidiasis (thrush) of the mouth, infected painful teeth and gums and excessive production of saliva. Also, for a sore infected throat, tonsillitis, mumps, discharging infected ear and a congested severe headache and pains in the joints. It is good for eye complaints including severe conjunctivitis, allergic conditions with a running nose, skin complaints that produce pus-filled pustules, spots and ulcers, including varicose ulcers. The symptoms are made worse by extremes of heat and cold and also for wet and rapidly changing weather. They are worse at night and for sweating and being too hot in bed.

Symptoms improve for rest and in comfortable temperatures where the person is neither too hot nor too cold. People suitable for mere. sol. tend to be very insecure although they have an outwardly calm appearance. They are cautious and reserved with other people and consider what they are about to say before speaking so that conversation may seem laboured. Mere, sol. types do not like criticism of any kind and may suddenly become angry if someone disagrees with their point of view. They tend to be introverted but their innermost thoughts may be in turmoil. They tend to be hungry and enjoy bread and butter, milk and other cold drinks but dislike alcohol with the exception of beer. They usually do not eat meat and do not have a sweet tooth. They dislike coffee and salt. Mere, sol. people often have fair hair with fine, unlined skin and an air of detachment. They are afraid of dying and of mental illness leading to insanity, and worry about the wellbeing of their family. They fear being burgled and are afraid or fearful during a thunderstorm.

Natrum muriaticum
Natrum mur; common salt, sodium chloride
Salt has long been prized for its seasoning and preservative qualities, and Roman soldiers were once paid in salt, such was its value. (Salary comes from the Latin word salarium, which refers to this practice). Sodium and chlorine are essential chemicals in the body, being needed for many metabolic processes, particularly the functioning of nerve tissue. In fact, there is seldom a need to add salt to food as usually enough is present naturally in a healthy, well-balanced diet. (An exception is when people are working very hard physically in a hot climate and losing a lot of salt in sweat). However, people and many other mammals frequently have a great liking for salt. If the salt/water balance in the body is disturbed, a person soon becomes very ill and may even die.

In ancient times, salt was usually obtained by boiling sea water, but natural evaporation around the shallow edges of salt lakes results in deposits of rock salt being formed. Rock salt is the usual source of table salt and also of the remedy used in homoeopathy. This remedy has an effect on the functioning of the kidneys and the salt/water balance of body fluids, and is used to treat both mental and physical symptoms. Emotional symptoms that benefit from natrum mur. include sensitivity and irritability, tearfulness and depression, suppressed grief and premenstrual tension. Physical ailments that respond to this remedy are often those in which there is a thin, watery discharge of mucus and in which symptoms are made worse by heat. Hence natrum mur. is used in the treatment of colds with a runny nose or other catarrhal problems. Also, for some menstrual and vaginal problems, headaches and migraines, cold sores, candidiasis (thrush) of the mouth, mouth ulcers, inflamed and infected gums and bad breath. Some skin disorders are helped by natrum mur. including verruca (a wart on the foot), warts, spots and boils and cracked, dry lips. It may be used in the treatment of fluid retention with puffiness around the face, eyelids and abdomen, etc, urine retention, constipation, anal fissure, indigestion, anaemia and thyroid disorders (goitre). When ill, people who benefit from this remedy feel cold and shivery but their symptoms are made worse, or even brought on, by heat. Heat, whether from hot sun and fire or a warm, stuffy room exacerbate the symptoms, which also are made worse in cold and thundery weather. They are worse on the coast from the sea breeze, and in the morning between 9 and 11 0' clock. Too much physical activity and the sympathy of others exacerbate the symptoms. They improve in the fresh, open air and for cold applications or a cold bath or swim. Also, sleeping on a hard bed and sweating and fasting make the symptoms better.

People suitable for natrum mur. are often women who are highly sensitive, serious-minded, intelligent and reliable. They have high ideals and feel things very deeply, being easily hurt and stung by slights and criticism. They need the company of other people but, being so sensitive, can actually shun them for fear of being hurt. They are afraid of mental illness leading to loss of self-control and insanity and of dying. Also, they fear the dark, failure in work, crowds, being burgled and have a tendency to be claustrophobic. They worry about being late and are fearful during a thunderstorm. Natrum. mur. people tend to become introverted and react badly to the criticism of others. They are highly sensitive to the influence of music, which easily moves them to tears. Natrum mur. people are usually of squat or solid build with dark or fairish hair. They are prone to reddened, watery eyes as though they have been crying, and a cracked lower lip. The face may appear puffy and shiny with an air of stoicism.

Nux vomica
Strychnos nux vomica; poison nut, Quaker buttons

The strychnos nux vomica tree is a native of India but also grows in Burma, Thailand, China and Australia. It produces small, greenish-white flowers and later, apple-sized fruits, containing small, flat, circular pale seeds covered in fine hair. The seeds, bark and leaves are highly poisonous, containing strychnine, and have been used in medicine for many centuries. In medieval times, the seeds were used as a treatment for the plague. Strychnine has severe effects upon the nervous system but in minute amounts can help increase urination and aid digestion. The seeds are cleaned and dried and used to produce the homoeopathic remedy. Nux vomica is used in the treatment of a variety of digestive complaints including cramping, colicky abdominal pains, indigestion, nausea and vomiting, diarrhoea and constipation. Also, indigestion or stomach upset caused by over-indulgence in alcohol or rich food and piles that cause painful contractions of the rectum. Sometimes, these complaints are brought on by a tendency to keep emotions, particularly anger, suppressed and not allowing it to show or be expressed outwardly. Nux vomica is a remedy for irritability, headache and migraine, colds, coughs and influenza-like symptoms offever, aching bones and muscles and chills and shivering. It is a useful remedy for women who experience heavy, painful periods that may cause fainting, morning sickness during pregnancy and pain in labour. It is also used to treat urinary frequency and cystitis.

The type of person who benefits from this remedy is frequently under stress and experiences a periodic flare-up of symptoms. The person may be prone to indigestion and heartburn, gastritis and stomach ulcer and piles or haemorrhoids. The person usually has a tendency to keep everything bottled up but has a passionate nature and is liable to outbursts of anger. Nux vomica people are very ambitious and competitive, demanding a high standard of themselves and others and intolerant of anything less than perfection. They enjoy challenges and using their wits to keep one step ahead. Often, they are to be found as managers, company directors, scientists, etc, at the cutting edge of their particular occupation. They are ungracious and irritable when ill and cannot abide the criticism of others. This type of person is afraid of being a failure at work and fears or dislikes crowded public places. He or she is afraid of dying. The person enjoys rich, fattening foods containing cholesterol and spicy meals, alcohol and coffee although these upset the digestive system. Symptoms are worse in cold, windy, dry weather and in winter and between 3 and 4 a.m. They are aggravated by certain noises, music, bright lights and touch, eating (especially spicy meals) and with overwork of mental faculties. Nux vomica people usually look serious, tense and are thin with a worried expression. They have sallow skin and tend to have dark shadows beneath the eyes.

Phosphorus
Phos; white phosphorus

Phosphorus is an essential mineral in the body, found in the genetical material (DNA), bones and teeth. White phosphorus is extremely flammable and poisonous and was once used in the manufacture of matches and fireworks. Due to the fact that it tends to catch fire spontaneously when exposed to air, it is stored under water. In the past it has been used to treat a number of disorders and infectious diseases such as measles. In homoeopathy, the remedy is used to treat nervous tension caused by stress and worry, with symptoms of sleeplessness, exhaustion and digestive upset. Often there are pains of a burning nature in the chest or abdomen. It is a remedy for vomiting and nausea, heartburn, acid indigestion, stomach ulcer and gastroenteritis. It is also used to treat bleeding, e.g. from minor wounds, the gums, nosebleeds, gastric and profuse menstrual bleeding.

Severe coughs that may be accompanied by retching, vomiting and production of a blood-tinged phlegm are treated with phos. as well as some other severe respiratory complaints. These include pneumonia, bronchitis, asthma and laryngitis. Styes that tend to recur and poor circulation may also be helped by phos. Symptoms are worse in the evening and morning and before or during a thunderstorm. They are also made worse for too much physical activity, hot food and drink and lying on the left side. Symptoms improve in the fresh open air and with lying on the back or right side. They are better after sleep or when the person is touched or stroked. People who need phos. do not like to be alone when ill and improve for the sympathy and attention of others. They are warm, kind, affectionate people who are highly creative, imaginative and artistic. They enjoy the company of other people and need stimulation to give impetus to their ideas. Phos. people have an optimistic outlook, are full of enthusiasm but sometimes promise much and deliver little. They are very tactile and like to be touched or stroked and offered sympathy when unhappy or unwell. They enjoy a variety of different foods but tend to suffer from digestive upsets. Phos. people are usually tall, slim and may be dark or fairhaired, with an attractive, open appearance. They like to wear brightly coloured clothes, and are usually popular, having many friends. They have a fear of illness, especially cancer, and of dying and also of the dark and supernatural forces. They are apprehensive of water and fear being a failure in their work. Thunderstorms make them nervous.

Pulsatilla nigricans
Pulsatilla; *Anemone pratensis*, meadow anemone

This attractive plant closely resembles *Anemone pulsatilla*, the pasque flower, which is used in herbal medicine, but has smaller flowers. *Anemone pratensis* is a native of Germany, Denmark and Scandinavia and has been used medicinally for hundreds of years. The plant produces beautiful deep purple flowers with orange centres and both leaves and flowers are covered with fine, silky hairs. The whole fresh plant is gathered and made into a pulp and liquid is extracted to make the remedy used in homoeopathy. It is used to treat a wide variety of disorders with both physical and mental symptoms. It is a useful remedy for ailments in which there is a greenish-yellowish discharge. Hence it is used for colds and coughs and sinusitis with the production of profuse catarrh or phlegm. Also, eye infections with discharge such as styes and conjunctivitis. Digestive disorders are helped by pulsatilla, particularly indigestion, heartburn, nausea and sickness caused by eating too much fatty or rich food. The remedy is helpful for female disorders in which there are a variety of physical and emotional symptoms. These include premenstrual tension, menstrual problems, menopausal symptoms and cystitis, with accompanying symptoms of mood swings, depression and tearfulness. It is a remedy for headaches and migraine, swollen glands, inflammation and pain in the bones and joints as in rheumatic and arthritic disorders, nosebleeds, varicose veins, mumps, measles, toothache, acne, frequent urination and incontinence.

Symptoms are worse at night or when it is hot, and after eating heavy, rich food. Symptoms improve out in the cool fresh air and with gentle exercise such as walking. The person feels better after crying and being treated sympathetically by others. Pulsatilla people are usually women who have a mild, passive nature and are kind, gentle and loving. They are easily moved to tears by the plight of others and love animals and people alike. The person yields easily to the requests and demands of others and is a peacemaker who likes to avoid a scene. An outburst of anger is very much out of character and a pulsatilla person usually has many friends. The person likes rich and sweet foods, although these may upset the digestion, and dislikes spicy meals. Pulsatilla people may fear darkness, being left alone, dying and any illness leading to insanity. They are fearful of crowds, the supernatural and tend to be claustrophobic. Usually, they are fair and blue-eyed with clear, delicate skin that blushes readily. They are attractive and slightly overweight or plump.

Sepia officinalis
Sepia; ink of the cuttlefish

Cuttlefish ink has been used since ancient times, both for medicinal purposes and as a colour in artists' paint. The cuttlefish has the ability to change colour to blend in with its surroundings and squirts out the dark brown/black ink when threatened by predators. Sepia was known to Roman physicians who used it as a cure for baldness. In homoeopathy it is mainly used as an excellent remedy for women experiencing menstrual and menopausal problems. It was investigated and proved by Hahnemann in 1834. It is used to treat premenstrual tension, menstrual pain and heavy bleeding, infrequent or suppressed periods, menopausal symptoms such as hot flushes and postnatal depression. Physical and emotional symptoms caused by an imbalance of hormones are helped by sepia. Also, conditions in which there is extreme fatigue or exhaustion with muscular aches and pains. Digestive complaints, including nausea and sickness, abdominal pain and wind, caused by eating dairy products, and headaches with giddiness and nausea are relieved by sepia. Also, it is a remedy for incontinence, hot, sweaty feet and verruca (a wart on the foot). A woman often experiences pelvic, dragging pains frequently associated with prolapsed of the womb. Disorders of the circulation, especially varicose veins and cold extremities benefit from sepia.

Symptoms are worse in cold weather and before a thunderstorm and in the late afternoon, evening and early in the morning. Also, before a period in women and if the person receives sympathy from others. The symptoms are better with heat and warmth, quick vigorous movements, having plenty to do and out in the fresh open air. People suitable for sepia are usually, but not exclusively, women. They tend to be tall, thin and with a yellowish complexion and are rather self-contained and indifferent to others. Sepia people may become easily cross, especially with family and close friends, and may harbour resentment. In company, they make a great effort to appear outgoing and love to dance. A woman may be either an externally hard, successful career person or someone who constantly feels unable to cope, especially with looking after the home and family. Sepia people have strongly held beliefs and cannot stand others taking a contrary opinion. When ill, they hate to be fussed over or have the sympathy of others. They like both sour and sweet foods and alcoholic drinks but are upset by milk products and fatty meals. They harbour deep insecurity and fear being left alone, illness resulting in madness and loss of their material possessions and wealth. One physical attribute is that they often have a brown mark in the shape of a saddle across the bridge of the nose.

Silicea terra
Silicea; silica.

Silica is one of the main rock-forming minerals and is also found in living things where its main function is to confer strength and resilience. In homoeopathy, it is used to treat disorders of the skin, nails and bones and recurring inflammations and infections, especially those that occur because the person is somewhat rundown or has an inadequate diet. Also, some disorders of the nervous
system are relieved by silicea. The homoeopathic remedy used to be derived from ground flint or quartz but is now prepared by chemical reaction. The remedy is used for catarrhal infections such as colds, influenza, sinusitis, ear infections including glue ear. Also, for inflammations producing pus such as a boil, carbuncle, abscess, stye, whitlow (infection of the finger nail) and peritonsillar abscess. It is beneficial in helping the natural expulsion of a foreign body such as a splinter in the skin. It is a remedy for a headache beginning at the back of the head and radiating forwards over the right eye and for stress-related conditions of over-work and sleeplessness.

Symptoms are worse for cold, wet weather, especially when clothing is inadequate, draughts, swimming and bathing, becoming chilled after removing clothes and in the morning. They are better for warmth and heat, summer weather, warm clothing, particularly a hat or head covering and not lying on the left side. People who are suitable for silicea tend to be thin with a fine build and pale skin. They often have thin, straight hair. They are prone to dry, cracked skin and nails and may suffer from skin infections. Silicea people are usually unassuming, and lacking in confidence and physical stamina. They are conscientious and hard-working to the point of working too hard once a task has been undertaken. However, they may hesitate to commit themselves through lack of confidence and fear of responsibility. Silicea people are tidy and obsessive about small details. They may feel 'put upon', but lack the courage to speak out, and may take this out on others who are not responsible for the situation. They fear failure and dislike exercise due to physical weakness, often feeling mentally and physically exhausted. They enjoy cold foods and drinks.

Sulphur
Sulphur; flowers of sulphur, brimstone.

Sulphur has a long history of use in medicine going back to very ancient times. Sulphur gives off sulphur dioxide when burnt, which smells unpleasant ('rotten eggs' odour) but acts as a disinfectant. This was used in medieval times to limit the spread of infectious diseases. Sulphur is deposited around the edges of hot springs and geysers and where there is volcanic activity. Flowers of sulphur, which is a bright yellow powder, is obtained from the natural mineral deposit and is used to make the homoeopathic remedy. Sulphur is found naturally in all body tissues and, in both orthodox medicine and homoeopathy, is used to treat skin disorders. It is a useful remedy for dermatitis, eczema, psoriasis and a dry, flaky, itchy skin or scalp. Some digestive disorders benefit from sulphur especially a tendency for food to rise back up to the mouth and indigestion caused by drinking milk. Sulphur is helpful in the treatment of haemorrhoids or piles, premenstrual and menopausal symptoms, eye inflammations such as conjunctivitis, pain in the lower part of the back, catarrhal colds and coughs, migraine headaches and feverish symptoms. Some mental symptoms are helped by this remedy particularly those brought about by stress or worry including depression, irritability, insomnia and lethargy. When ill, people who benefit from sulphur feel thirsty rather than hungry and are upset by unpleasant smells. The person soon becomes exhausted and usually sleeps poorly at night and is tired through the day. The symptoms are worse in cold, damp conditions, in the middle of the morning around 11 a.m. and in stuffy, hot, airless rooms. Also, for becoming too hot at night in bed and for wearing too many layers of clothes. Long periods of standing and sitting aggravate the symptoms and they are worse if the person drinks alcohol or has a wash. Symptoms improve in dry, clear, warm weather and for taking exercise. They are better if the person lies on the right side.

Sulphur people tend to look rather untidy and have dry, flaky skin and coarse, rough hair. They may be thin, round-shouldered and inclined to slouch or be overweight, round and red-faced. Sulphur people have lively, intelligent minds full of schemes and inventions, but are often useless on a practical level. They may be somewhat self-centred with a need to be praised, and fussy over small unimportant details. They enjoy intellectual discussion on subjects that they find interesting and may become quite heated although the anger soon subsides. Sulphur people are often warm and generous with their time and money. They enjoy a wide range of foods but are upset by milk and eggs. They have a fear of being a failure in their work, of heights and the supernatural.

Additional homoeopathic medicines in common use

Aconitum nepalese (aconite, monkshood, wolfsbane, friar's cap, mousebane)
Actea racemosa (black snakeroot, rattleroot, bugbane, rattleweed, squaw root)
Allium (Spanish onion)

Apis mellifica (the honey bee)

Arnica montana (arnica; leopard's bane, sneezewort)

Atropa belladonna (belladonna; deadly nightshade, black cherry, devil's cherries, naughty man's cherries, de vil's herb)

Aurum metallicum (aurum met; gold)

Bryonia alba (bryonia; European white bryony, black-berried white bryony, wild hops)

Calcarea fluorica (calc. fluor; fluorite, calcium fluoride, fluoride of lime)

Calcarea phosphorica (calc. phos; phosphate of lime, calcium phosphate)

Calendula officinalis (calendula; marigold, garden marigold)

Cantharis vesicatoria (cantharis; Spanish fly)

Carbo vegetablis (carbo veg; vegetable charcoal)

Chamomilla (chamomile; common chamomile, double chamomile)

China officinalis (cinchona succiruba; china, Peruvian bark, Jesuit's bark)

Citrullus colocynthus (colocynthis; bitter cucumber, bitter apple)

Cuprum metallicum (cuprum met; copper)

Daphne mezereum (daphne; spurge laurel, wild pepper, spurge olive, flowering spurge, dwarf bay)

Drosera rotundi folia (drosera; sundew, youthwort, red rot, moor grass)

Euphrasia officinalis (euphrasia; eyebright)

Ferrum phosphoricum (ferrum phos; phosphate of iron, iron phosphate)

Gelsemium sempervirens (gelsemium; yellow jasmine, false jasmine, Carolina jasmine, wild woodbine)

Guaiacum offinale (guaiac; resin of lignum vitae)

Hamamelis virginiana hamamelis (witch hazel; spotted alder, snapping hazelnut, winterbloom)

Hepar sulphuris calcareum (hepar sulph; sulphide of calcium)

Hypericum perforatum (hypericum, St John's wort)

Ipecacuanha (ipecac; cephalis ipecacuanha, psychotria ipecacuanha, the ipecac plant)

Kalium bichromicum (kali bich; potassium dichromate, potassium bichromate)

Kalium iodatum (kali iod; kali hydriodicum, potassium iodide)

Kalium phosphoricum (kali phos; potassium phosphate, phosphate of potash)

Ledum palustre (ledum: marsh tea, wild rosemary)

Rhus toxicodendron (rhus tox; rhus radicaris, American poison ivy, poison oak, poison vine)

Ruta graveolens (ruta grav; rue, garden rue, herbygrass, ave-grace, herb-of-grace, bitter herb)

Tarentula cubensis (tarentula cub; Cuban tarentula)

Thuja occidentalis (thuja; tree of life, yellow cedar, arbor vitae, false white cedar)

Urtica urens (urtica; stinging nettle)

Glossary of terms used in homoeopathy

aggravations a term first used by Dr Samuel Hahnemann to describe an initial worsening of symptoms experienced by some patients, on first taking a homoeopathic remedy, before the condition improved. In modern homoeopathy this is known as a'healing crisis'. To prevent the occurrence of aggravations, Hahnemann experimented with further dilutions of remedies and, in particular, vigorous shaking (succussing) of preparations at each stage of the process.

allopathy a term first used by Or Samuel Hahnemann meaning 'against disease'. It describes the approach of conventional medicine, which is to treat symptoms with a substance or drug with an opposite effect in order to suppress or eliminate them. This is called the Law of Contraries and is in direct contrast to the 'like can cure like,' the Law of Similars or *Similia Similibus Curentur* principle, which is central to the practice of homoeopathy.

centesimal scale of dilution the scale of dilution used in homoeopathy based on one part (or drop) of the remedy in 99 parts of the diluents liquid (a mixture of alcohol and water).

classical the practice of homoeopathy based on the work of Or Samuel Hahnemann and further developed and expanded by other practitioners, particularly Or Constantine Hering and Or lames Tyler Kent.

constitutional prescribing and constitutional types the homoeopathic concept, based on the work of Or lames Tyler Kent, that prescribing should be based on the complete make-up of a person, including physical and emotional characteristics, as well as on the symptoms of a disorder.

decimal scale of dilution the scale of dilution used in homoeopathy based on one part (or drop) of the remedy in nine parts of the diluents liquid (a mixture of alcohol and water).

healing crisis the situation in which a group of symptoms first become worse after a person has taken a homoeopathic remedy, before they improve and disappear. The occurrence of a healing crisis is taken to indicate a change and that improvement is likely to follow. It is usually short-lived, *(see also aggravations)*.

homoeopathy the system of healing based on the principle of 'like can cure like' and given its name by Samuel Hahnemann. The word is derived from the Greek *homeo* for similar and *pathos* for suffering, or 'like disease'.

laws of cure, law of direction of cure three concepts or 'laws' formulated by Dr Constantine Hering to explain the means by which symptoms of disease are eliminated from the body in homoeopathy.

I. Symptoms move in a downwards direction.

2. Symptoms move from the inside of the body outwards.
3. Symptoms move from more important vital organs and tissues to those of less importance.

Hering was also responsible for the view in homoeopathy that more recent symptoms disappear first before ones that have been present for a longer time. Hence symptoms are eliminated in the reverse order of their appearance.

materia medica detailed information about homoeopathic remedies, listed alphabetically and includes details of the symptoms that may respond to each remedy, based on previous research and experience. Details about the source of each remedy are also included. This information is used by a homoeopathic doctor when deciding upon the best remedy for each particular patient and group of symptoms.

miasm a chronic constitutional weakness that is the after-effect of an underlying suppressed disease that has been present in a previous generation or earlier in the life of an individual. The concept of miasm was formulated by Samuel Hahnemann who noted that some people were never truly healthy but always acquired new symptoms of illness. He believed that this was due to a constitutional weakness that he called a miasm, which may have been inherited and was caused by an illness in a previous generation. These theories were put forward in his research writings entitled *Chronic Diseases.* Three main miasms were identified, psora, sycosis and syphilis.

modalities a term applied to the responses of the patient, when he or she feels better or worse, depending upon factors in the internal and external environment. These are unique from one person to another depending upon the individual characteristics that apply at the time, although there are common features within each constitutional type. Modalities include responses, fears and preferences to temperature, weather, foods, emotional responses and relationships, etc, which all contribute to a person's total sense of wellbeing. Modalities are particularly important when a person has symptoms of an illness in prescribing the most beneficial remedy.

mother tincture (symbol 0) the first solution obtained from dissolving a substance in a mixture of alcohol and water (usually in the ratio of 9/10 pure alcohol to 1/10 distilled water). The mother tincture is subjected to further dilutions and succussions (shakings) to produce the homoeopathic remedies.

nosode a term used to describe a remedy prepared from samples of infected diseased tissue, often to treat or prevent a particular illness. They were first investigated by Wilhelm Lux, not without considerable controversy. Examples are *Medorrhinum and Tuberculinum.*

organon *The Organon of Rationale Medicine.* One of the most important works of Samuel Hahnemann, published in Leipzig in 1810, in which he set out the principles and philosophy of modern homoeopathy. The *Organon* is considered to be a classic work and basic to the study of homoeopathy.

polycrest a remedy suitable for a number of illnesses, disorders or symptoms.

potency the dilution or strength of a homoeopathic remedy. Dr Samuel Hahnemann discovered that by further diluting and succussing (shaking) a remedy, it became more effective or potent in bringing about a cure. It is held that the process of diluting and shaking a remedy releases its innate energy or dynamism, even though none of the original molecules of the substance may remain. Hence the greater the dilution of a remedy, the stronger or more potent it becomes. Hahnemann called his new dilute solutions 'potentizations'.

potentiate the release or transfer of energy into a homoeopathic solution by succussing or vigorous shaking)f the mixture.

principle of vital force 'vital force' was the term given by Samuel Hahnemann to the inbuilt power or ability of the human body to maintain health and fitness and to fight off illness. Illness is believed to be the result of stresses that cause an imbalance in the vital force, and assail all people throughout life and include inherited, environmental and emotional factors. The symptom of this 'disorder' is illness, and this is held to be the physical indication of the struggle of the body's vital force to regain its balance. A person with a strong vital force will tend to remain in good health and to fight off illness. A person with a weak vital force is more likely to suffer from long-term, recurrent symptoms and illnesses. Homoeopathic remedies are believed to act upon the vital force, stimulating it to heal the body and restore the natural balance.

provings the term given by Samuel Hahnemann to experimental trials he carried out to test the reactions of healthy people to homoeopathic substances. 'these trials were carried out under strictly controlled conditions (in advance of the modern scientific approach), and the symptoms produced were meticulously recorded. Quinine was the substance that Hahnemann first investigated in this way, testing it initially on himself and then on close friends and family members. He continued over the next few years to investigate and prove many other substances, building up a wealth of information on each one about the reactions and symptoms it produced. After conducting this research, Hahnemann went on carefully to prescribe the remedies to those who were sick. Provings are still carried out in modern homoeopathy to test new substances that may be of value as remedies. Usually, neither the prescribing physician nor those taking the substance-the 'provers' -know the identity of the material or whether they are taking a placebo.

psora one of three miasms identified by Samuel Hahnemann believed to be caused by suppression of scabies. Psora was believed to have an inherited element or to be caused by suppression of an earlier infection in a particular individual.

Schussler tissue salts Wilhelm Heinrich Schussler was a German homoeopathic doctor who introduced the Biochemic Tissue Salt system in the late 1800s. Schussler believed that many symptoms and ailments resulted from the lack of a minute, but essential, quantity of a mineral or tissue salt. He identified twelve such tissue salts that he regarded as essential and believed that a cure could be obtained from replacing the deficient substance. Schussler's work was largely concentrated at the cell and tissue level rather than embracing the holistic view of homoeopathy.

similia similibus curentur the founding principle of homoeopathy that 'like can cure like' or 'let like be treated by like', which was first put forward by Hippocrates, a physician of ancient Greece. This principle excited the interest of Paracelsus in the Middle Ages, and was later restated and put into practice by Samuel Hahnemann with the development of homoeopathy.

similiimum a homoeopathic remedy that in its natural state is able to produce the same symptoms as those being exhibited by the patient.

succussion vigorous shaking of a homoeopathic remedy at each stage of dilution, along with banging the container and holding it against a hard surface, therebycausing further release of energy.

sycosis one of the three major miasms identified by Samuel Hahnemann and believed to result from a suppressed gonorrhoeal infection. Sycosis was believed to have an inherited element or to be due to suppression of an earlier infection in a particular individual. syphilis the third of the three major miasms identified by Samuel Hahnemann believed to result from a suppressed syphilis infection.

Syphilis was believed to have an inherited element or to be due to suppression of an earlier infection in a particular individual.

Trituration the process, devised by Samuel Hahnemann, of rendering naturally insoluble substances soluble so that they can be made available as homoeopathic remedies. The process involves repeated grinding down of the substance with lactose powder until it becomes soluble. The substance usually becomes soluble at the third process of trituration. Each trituration is taken to be the equivalent of one dilution in the centesimal scale. Once the substance has been rendered soluble, dilution can proceed in the normal way.

Hydrotherapy

Hydrotherapy is the use of water to heal and ease a variety of ailments, and the water may be used in a number of different ways. The healing properties of water have been recognized since ancient times, notably by the Greek, Roman and Turkish civilizations but also by people in Europe and China. Most people know the benefits of a hot bath in relaxing the body, relieving muscular aches and stiffness, and helping to bring about restful sleep. Hot water or steam causes blood vessels to dilate, opens skin pores and stimulates perspiration, and relaxes limbs and muscles. A cold bath or shower acts in the opposite way and is refreshing and invigorating. The cold causes blood vessels in the skin to constrict and blood is diverted to internal tissues and organs to maintain the core temperature of the body. Applications of cold water or ice reduce swelling and bruising and cause skin pores to close.

Treatment techniques in hydrotherapy

Hot baths are used to ease muscle and joint pains and inflammation. Also, warm or hot baths, with the addition of various substances such as seaweed extract to the water, may be used to help the healing of some skin conditions or minor wounds. After childbirth, frequent bathing in warm water to which a mild antiseptic has been added is recommended to heal skin tears.

Cold baths are used to improve blood flow to internal tissues and organs and to reduce swellings. The person may sit for a moment in shallow cold water with additional water being splashed onto exposed skin. An inflamed, painful part may be immersed in cold water to reduce swelling. The person is not allowed to become chilled, and this form of treatment is best suited for those able to dry themselves rapidly with a warm towel. It is not advisable for people with serious conditions or for the elderly or very young.

Steam baths, along with saunas and Turkish baths, are used to encourage sweating and the opening of skin pores and have a cleansing and refreshing effect. The body may be able to eliminate harmful
substances in this way and treatment finishes with a cool bath.

Sitz baths are usually given as a treatment for painful conditions with broken skin, such as piles or anal fissure, and also for ailments affecting the urinary and genital organs. The person sits in a specially designed bath that has two compartments, one with warm water, the other with cold. First, the person sits in the warm water, which covers the lower abdomen and hips, with the feet in the cold water compartment. After three minutes, the patient changes round and sits in the cold water with the feet in the warm compartment.

Hot and cold sprays of water may be given for a number of different disorders but are not recommended for those with serious illnesses, elderly people or young children.

Wrapping is used for feverish conditions, backache and bronchitis. A cold wet sheet that has been squeezed out is wrapped around the person, followed by a dry sheet and warm blanket. These are left in place until the inner sheet has dried and the coverings are then removed. The body is sponged with tepid water (at blood heat) before being dried with a towel. Sometimes the wrap is applied to a smaller area of the body, such as the lower abdomen, to ease a particular problem, usually constipation.

In orthodox medicine, hydrotherapy is used as a technique of physiotherapy for people recovering from serious injuries with problems of muscle wastage. Also, it is used for people with joint problems and those with severe physical disabilities. Many hospitals also offer the choice of a water birth to expectant mothers, and this has become an increasingly popular method of childbirth. Hydrotherapy may be offered as a form of treatment for other medical conditions in naturopathy, using the techniques listed above. It is wise to obtain medical advice before proceeding with hydrotherapy, and this is especially important for elderly persons, children and those with serious conditions or illnesses.

Hypnotherapy

The word hypnotherapy is based on the term hypnosis, which is derived from the Greek word hypnos meaning 'sleep'. The word hypnosis was invented in the 19th century by lames Braid, a Scottish surgeon, who sometimes used the technique of mesmerism while performing operations. He was not the only doctor to practise hypnotism at that time. In India, lames Esdaile used it as the sole anaesthetic for many operations. This was in complete contravention to medical opinion at that time, since for over 50 years the practice and theory of mesmerism had been condemned.

Mesmerism originated with Dr Franz Mesmer (1734-1815) who became convinced, from his research into the power and use of magnets, that magnetism existed as an unseen fluid that passed through and joined everything in the world. Magnets and powers of hypnosis seem to have been used for centuries whether in ancient Greece, by medicine men and witch doctors or by priests.
Mesmer believed that illness was precipitated when this force did not flow freely and that to cure ailments, the use of magnets was necessary to correct the flow. For a time his popularity increased in his practice in Vienna, but when unsuccessful cases occurred, he was criticized by the University and forced to leave the city.

After moving to Paris in 1778 he again found fame by having a clientele who came for the theatrical atmosphere and effects as well as to be cured. His patients were put into a trance by the combination of soft lights and music as they stood holding on to a container that held iron filings and water. Dr Mesmer maintained that they then received the effects of the 'magnetism' while he held a rod made of iron. It is now thought that his strong personality, charisma and powers of suggestion were the source of any cures, with his patients actually being 'mesmerised'. After investigation by the French medical profession and establishment, no scientific basis to his practice was found. They also did not approve of the methods he used and were aware of the scandal connected with his name. As a result his methods faded into obscurity.

With the advent of new anaesthetics such as chloroform and ether, the technique of hypnotherapy fell out of use, although it was obvious that it could successfully deaden pain. Around the) 900s, hypnotism was again investigated by the British Medical Association, but approval was not forthcoming. It has only recently regained some popularity with hypnotherapists viewing the trance as a condition in which body and mind can be calm and serene. While in this state, alterations can be made that are not achievable while the patient is completely conscious. The state of being neither fully awake nor fully asleep can be compared to when a person is 'miles away', i.e. daydreaming, or to a person who is sleepwalking. Whilst in a trance a person can function correctly and carry out tasks, converse sensibly and carry out requests. Unlike a sleep-walker, a person in a trance is open to requests or suggestions from the therapist. Both mental or physical changes can be effected, such as the lessening of pain, healing disorders and encouraging relaxation. Sometimes, a patient may have a problem that originates with an event that happened some time ago, e.g. in their childhood. If this is the case, and the patient can be helped to accept what has happened in the past through the use of hypnotherapy, this can also boost morale and self-confidence.

The aim of hypnotherapy is that the patient and therapist work together to achieve a cure. There is a variety of disorders that have been treated with success, such as migraine, irritable bowel syndrome, ulcers and skin disorders along with other problems caused by stress and anxiety. Illnesses known as hysterical illness are a relatively common problem that hypnotherapists treat. They include phobias (a fear of flying, heights, etc), insomnia and asthma. The pain of childbirth can also be relieved.

To ensure that any hypnotherapist is fully trained, it is advisable to contact the relevant professional organization. As well as the hypnotherapist being fully trained, a patient must feel that they can trust and talk openly to their therapist on personal matters, if need be. The nature and character of the therapist is therefore also extremely important so that the two can work together to alleviate the problem. The cost of private sessions, and the number needed can vary considerably although on average it is likely to be between five and ten, depending on the condition being treated. Consultations may differ in manner from one therapist to another but detailed case notes will be taken including all relevant treatments, both past and current, and any other information that it is felt might be relevant to the problem. Each session will last from approximately 30minutes to) hour. It is not usual for hypnosis to be used at the first consultation although a patient's reaction to it may be assessed. The patient should also be fully informed as to the content of each session and should be prepared to cooperate with the therapist in any discussion as to the aim of the treatment.

To induce a trance, a patient will be asked to concentrate their attention on a fixed object or something that is moving slowly, and this will encourage the patient to become drowsy. Whilst at this level of consciousness, the therapist is able to encourage the patient to view any problem more positively, to realize what they can achieve and also to understand any events in their past history and how they might be likely to react in the future. It is quite unusual for a patient to actually go to sleep after they have been in a trance. Should this happen it only demonstrates that the person has not had sufficient sleep and is merely tired. It is quite commonplace for a patient to use hypnosis on themselves after the ailment or problem, such as insomnia or asthma, has been resolved. With a little daily practice, they will be able to help themselves considerably should the need arise for further or frequent treatment. To assist the patient, a therapist might provide a pre-recorded tape of the known commencement of each session, which leads up to the trance.

The following example shows how a person could overcome a fear of flying. At the first visit to the hypnotherapist, once in a trance, the patient was told to imagine travelling and arriving at an airport. At the second and subsequent visits, the person gradually imagined the stages of boarding an aeroplane, going on a very short flight and finally travelling to a different country. To help the patient afterwards, a recording of the consultations had been made and these could be played in the home whenever required. The treatment proved to be completely successful with the patient being able to fly overseas frequently.

It is considered advisable to consult a hypnotherapist who is qualified as a general practitioner too, since should there be any specific disease present it will be recognized as such. Not all doctors are convinced that there is a scientific foundation for hypnosis, but for those who are also qualified hypnotherapists, the practice is incorporated with conventional treatments. Once a person is in a trance and past events have been brought to mind, other bodily functions such as brain activity and the pulse rate will react as if the event was actually happening. When a person in a trance imagines themselves to be a very young baby and the foot is stroked gently underneath, the reflex action is for the toes to curl upwards. This is the reflex response of a baby under six months old, after which the toes no longer curl upwards but downwards. This demonstrates how the person actually regresses to being very young and with the reflex actions applicable to that age.

Although aware of the existence of this sort of evidence, doubt has been expressed by some doctors that people are actually put into a trance. They tend to believe that there are different sorts of consciousness, with the level related to reality ceasing to work and another level taking control that is associated more with the imaginative and perceptive part of the mind. When fully conscious, the normal reaction would be to reject any thoughts or suggestions placed whilst under the influence of hypnosis. Concern has been expressed that a patient's memories of past events have been slightly modified or altered in some way to become what the patient or therapist would want them to be. Although these uncertainties about the trance state do exist, it is still recognized that hypnotherapy provides relief from pain without the use of drugs and is valuable in the treatment of various psychosomatic disorders.

Kinesiology

Kinesiology is a method of maintaining health by ensuring that all muscles are functioning correctly. It is believed that each muscle is connected with a specific part of the body such as the digestive system, circulation of the blood and specific organs, and if a muscle is not functioning correctly this will cause a problem in its related part of the body. The word is derived from kinesis, which is Greek for 'motion'. Kinesiology originated in 1964 and was developed by an American chiropractor named George Goodheart who realized that while he was treating a patient for severe pain in the leg, by massaging a particular muscle in the upper leg, the pain experienced by the patient eased and the muscle was strengthened.

Although he used the same method on different muscles, the results were not the same. Previous research done by an osteopath named Dr Chapman, in the 1900s, indicated that there were certain 'pressure points' in the body that were connected with particular muscles and, if these were massaged, lymph would be able to flow more freely through the body. Using these pressure points, Chapman found which point was connected to each particular muscle and realized why, when he had massaged a patient's upper leg muscle, the pain had lessened. The pressure point for that leg muscle was the only one that was situated above the actual muscle-all the other points were not close to the part of the body with which they were connected.

In the 1930s it was claimed that there were similar 'pressure points' located on the skull and, by exerting a light pressure on these, the flow of blood to their related organs could be assisted. Goodheart tested this claim, which originated from an osteopath called Terence Bennett, and discovered that after only fingertip pressure for a matter of seconds, it improved the strength of a particular muscle. After some time he was able to locate sixteen points on the head, the back of the knee and by the breastbone that were all allied to groups of important muscles. Goodheart was surprised that so little force applied on the pressure point could have such an effect on the muscle, so to further his studies he then applied himself to acupuncture. This is a form of healing that also makes use of certain points located over the body but that run along specific paths known as meridians. After further study, Goodheart came to the conclusion that the meridians could be used for both muscles and organs. The invisible paths used in kinesiology are exactly the same as the ones for acupuncture.

A kinesiologist will examine a patient and try to discover whether there is any lack of energy, physical disorders or inadequate nutrition that is causing problems. Once any troublesome areas have been located, the practitioner will use only a light massage on the relevant pressure points (which, as mentioned, are generally not close to their associated muscle). For example, the edge of the rib cage is where the pressure points for the muscles of the upper leg are situated. In kinesiology it is maintained that the use of pressure points is effective because the flow of blood to muscles is stimulated and therefore a good supply of lymph is generated too. Lymph is a watery fluid that takes toxins from the tissues and if muscles receive a good supply of both lymph and blood they should function efficiently. As in acupuncture, it is maintained that there is an unseen flow of energy that runs through the body and if this is disrupted for any reason, such as a person being ill or suffering from stress, then the body will weaken due to insufficient energy being produced. The way in which a kinesiologist assesses the general health of a patient is by testing the strength of the muscles as this will provide information on the flow of energy. It is claimed that by finding any imbalance and correcting it, kinesiology can be used as a preventive therapy. If there is a lack of minerals and vitamins in the body or trouble with the digestive system, it is claimed that these are able to be diagnosed by the use of kinesiology. If a person is feeling 'below par' and constantly feels tired, it is believed that these conditions are aggravated by a sluggish flow of the internal body fluids such as the circulation of blood. Kinesiologists can treat the disorder by stimulating the flow of lymph and blood by massaging the pressure points.

Although it is claimed that kinesiology can be of help to all people, it is widely known for the treatment of people suffering from food allergies or those who are sensitive to some foods. It is believed that the chemicals and nutrients contained in food cause various reactions in the body, and if a particular food has the effect of making muscles weak, then it would be concluded that a person has an allergy to it. Allergic reactions can cause other problems such as headaches, tension, colds, tiredness and a general susceptibility to acquiring any passing infections.

There are two simple tests that can easily be tried at home to determine if there is any sensitivity or allergy to certain foods. This is done by testing the strength of a strong muscle in the chest, and to carry this out the person being tested will need the help of a partner. There is no need to exert real force at any time, just use the minimum amount needed to be firm but gentle. To test the chest muscle, sit erect, holding the left arm straight out at right angles to the body. The elbow should be facing outwards and the fingers and thumb drooping towards the table. The partner will then place his or her right hand on the person's nearest shoulder (the right) and the two fingers only on the area around the left wrist. A gentle downward pressure will then be exerted by the partner on the person's wrist who will try to maintain the level of the arm, whilst breathing in a normal fashion. This downward pressure should be exerted for approximately five seconds. If the person was able to resist the downwards pressure and the muscle felt quite firm, then the allergy test can be tried. However, if this was not the case and the person was unable to keep the arm level, the muscle would not be suitable for use in the subsequent test. It would therefore be advisable to use another muscle such as one in the arm. To do this, place an arm straight down at the side of the body with the palm of the hands facing outwards. The partner will then use the same amount of pressure to try and move the arm outwards, again for a similar amount of time. If the person is unable to keep the arm in the same position, then it would be advisable to get in touch with a trained kinesiologist. To undertake the allergy test, hold the left arm in the same way as for testing the muscle. If, for example, the food that is suspected of causing an allergy is chocolate, a small piece of this should be put just in the mouth, there is no need for ii to be eaten. This time as well as applying the pressure on the wrist as before, the partner should put his or her first two digits of the left hand below the person's right ear. Once again, the person tries to resist the downwards force and if successful, it is claimed that there is no sensitivity or allergy connected with that food. However, if this does not happen and the arm is pushed downwards or even feels slightly weak, then kinesiology would suggest that this food, if eaten at all, should never be consumed in any great amount.

It is claimed that the use of kinesiology can be of benefit to people who suffer from irrational fears or phobias. An example of this is the recommendation that the bone below the eye, just level with the pupil, is softly tapped. Neck and back pain can be treated without any manipulation of joints and some of the methods can be learnt by patients for use at home. An example of this for the alleviation of back pain is for a patient to massage the muscle situated on the inside of the thigh. This is said to be of benefit for any muscles that are weak as they are the reason for a painful back.

A number of other practitioners, such as homoeopaths, herbalists and osteopaths make use of kinesiology, so if there is a problem connected with the ligaments, muscles or bones it may be advisable to contact a chiropractor or osteopath who is also qualified in kinesiology. If the problem is of a more emotional or mental nature, then it might be best to select a counsellor or psychotherapist who also practises kinesiology. It is important always to use a fullyqualified practitioner and the relevant association should be contacted for information. At the first consultation, detailed questions will be asked concerning the medical history, followed by the therapist checking the muscles' ability to function effectively.

For instance, a slight pressure will be exerted on a leg or arm while the patient holds it in a certain way. The patient's ability to maintain that position against the pressure is noted and if the patient is unable to do so, then the therapist will find the reason why by further examination. Once the areas in need of 'rebalancing' have been identified, the therapist will use the relevant pressure points to correct matters. It is believed that if some of the points are painful or sore to the touch, this is because there has been an accumulation of toxins in the tissues, and these toxins stop the impulses between muscles and the brain. If this is the case, the muscle is unable to relax properly and can cause problems in areas such as the neck and shoulders.

There are ways of identifying any possible problems. For example, if there is any weakness in the shoulder muscle it may be that there is some problem connected with the lungs. To test for this, the patient sits upright with one arm raised to slightly below shoulder level and the other arm lower and out to the front. The therapist grasps the patient's upper arm and presses gently downwards on the raised arm at the elbow. If the muscle is functioning correctly then this downwards force should not be allowed to move the arm lower. If the patient is suffering from pain in the back. the probable cause lies with weak muscles in the stomach. To test for this. the patient sits on the floor with the knees raised. the arms crossed on the chest and then they lean backwards. The therapist checks the stomach muscles' efficiency by pushing gently backwards on the patient's crossed arms. If all is well the patient should be able to maintain the position and not lean back any further.

After treatment by massage of the pressure points. there may well be some tenderness experienced for one or two days as the toxins in the tissues dissipate gradually. However. there should be an overall feeling of an improvement in health and in particular with the problem that was being treated.

Although there has been an increase in the use of kinesiology by doctors to help discover the cause of an ailment. there has been little scientific research carried out. Therefore. the majority of doctors using conventional medicine do not believe that the flow of electrical energy present in the body can be changed by the use of massage or similar methods.

Massage

As long ago as 3000 BC massage was used as a therapy in the
Far East, making it one of the oldest treatments used by
humans. In 5 BC in ancient Greece, Hippocrates recommended
that to maintain health a massage using oils should be taken
daily after a perfumed bath. The physicians there were well
used to treating people who suffered from pain and stiffness in
the joints.

Massage increased in popularity when, in the 19th century, Per
Henrik Ling, a Swedish athlete, created the basis for what is now
known as Swedish massage. Swedish massage is a combination
of relaxing effects and exercises that work on the joints and
muscles, but it is still based on the form that was practised in
ancient times. More recently, a work was published by George
Downing in the 1970s called *The Massage Book,* and this
introduced a new concept in the overall technique of massage,
that the whole person's state should be assessed by the
therapist and not solely the
physical side. The emotional and mental states should be part of
the overall picture. Also combined in his form of massage were
the methods used in reflexology and shiatsu, and this was
known
as therapeutic massage. The aim of this is to use relaxation,
stimulation and invigoration to promote good health.

This massage is commonly used to induce general relaxation, so
that any tension or strain experienced in the rush of daily life
can be eased and eliminated. It is found to be very effective,
working on the mind as well as the body. It can be used to treat
people with hypertension (high blood pressure), sinusitis,
headaches, insomnia and hyperactivity, including people who
suffer from heart ailments or circulatory disorders. At the
physical level, massage is intended to help the body make use
of food and to eliminate the waste materials, as well as
stimulating the nervous and muscular system and the

circulation of blood. Neck and back pain are conditions from which many people suffer, particularly if they have not been sitting correctly, such as in a slightly stooped position with their shoulders rounded. People whose day-to-day work involves a great deal of physical activity, such as dancers and athletes, can also derive a great deal of benefit from the use of massage.

Stiffness can be a problem that they have after training or working, and this is relieved by encouraging the toxins that gather in the muscles to disperse. Massage promotes a feeling of calmness and serenity, and this is particularly beneficial to people who frequently suffer from bouts of depression or anxiety. Once the worry and depression have been dispelled, people are able to deal with their problems much more effectively and, being able to do so, will boost their self-confidence.

In hospitals, massage has been used to ease pain and discomfort as well as being of benefit to people who are bedridden, since the flow of blood to the muscles is stimulated. It has also been used for those who have suffered a heart attack and has helped their recovery. A more recent development has been the use of massage for cancer patients who are suffering from the after-effects of treatment, such as chemotherapy, as well as the discomfort the disease itself causes. Indeed, there are few conditions when it is not recommended. However, it should not be used when people are suffering from inflammation of the veins (phlebitis), varicose veins, thrombosis (clots in the blood) or if they have a raised temperature such as occurs during a fever. It is then advisable to contact a doctor before using massage. Doctors may be able to recommend a qualified therapist, a health centre may be able to help or contact can be made with the relevant professional body.

It is quite usual nowadays for a masseur or masseuse to combine treatment with the use of other methods, such as aromatherapy, acupuncture or reflexology. Massage can be divided into four basic forms, and these are known as *percussion* (also known as drumming); friction (also called pressure); *effleurage* (also called stroking) and *petrissage* (also called kneading). These four methods can be practised alone or in combination for maximum benefit to problems with damaged ligaments or tendons. This is because the flow of blood is stimulated and the movement of joints is improved. Friction can be performed with the base of the hand, some fingers or the upper part of the thumb. It is not advisable to use this method on parts of the body that have been injured in some way, for example where there is bruising.

Effleurage is performed in a slow, controlled manner using both hands together with a small space between the thumbs. If the therapist wishes to use only light pressure he or she will use the palms of the hands or the tips of the fingers, whilst for increased pressure the knuckles or thumbs will be used. Massage is a therapy in which both parties derive an overall feeling of wellbeing-the therapist by the skilful use of the hands to impart the relaxation, and the patient through the therapy being administered.

Percussion is also called tapotement, which is derived from *tapoter,* a French word that means 'to drum', as of the fingers on a surface. As would be expected from its name, percussion is generally
done with the edge of the hand with a quick, chopping movement, although the strokes are not hard. This type of movement would be used on places like the buttocks, thighs, waist or shoulders
where there is a wide expanse of flesh.

Friction is often used on dancers and athletes who experience *Petrissage* employs a kneading action on parts of a muscle. As the therapist works across each section, an area of flesh is grasped and squeezed, and this action stimulates the flow of blood and enables tensed muscles to relax. People such as athletes can have an accumulation of lactic acid in certain muscles, and this is why cramp occurs. Parts of the body on which this method is practised are along the stomach and around the waist.

A session may be undertaken in the patient's home, or he or she can attend the masseur or masseuse at a clinic. At each session the client will undress, leaving only pants or briefs on, and will lie on a firm, comfortable surface, such as a table that is designed especially for massage. The massage that follows normally lasts from 20 minutes to one hour. Women in labour have found that the pain experienced during childbirth can be eased if massage is performed on the buttocks and back. The massage eases the build-up of tension in the muscles, encouraging relaxation and easing of labour pains. It is said to be more effective on women who had previously experienced the benefits and reassurance of massage.

For anyone who is competent and wishes to provide some simple massage for a partner, there are some basic rules to follow. The room should be warm and peaceful. The surface on which the person lies is quite comfortable but firm. A futon (a quilted Japanese mattress) can be used, and to relieve the upper part of the body from any possible discomfort, a pillow should be placed underneath the torso. Any pressure that may be exerted on the feet can be dispelled by the use of a rolled-up towel or similar placed beneath the ankles. Both people should be relaxed, and to this end soft music can be played. All the movements of the hand should be of a continuous nature. It is suggested that the recipient always has one hand of the masseur or masseuse placed on him or her.

Vegetable oil (about one teaspoonful) is suitable but should not be poured straight on to the person. It should be spread over the hands by rubbing, which will also warm it sufficiently for use. Should the masseur or masseuse get out of breath, he or she should stop for a rest, all the while retaining a hand on the person.

Massage of the head and face begins with the forehead, which should be massaged using the thumbs. This is done by stroking them outwards from the centre across the forehead. This can also be repeated for the cheeks. The jaw line can then be squeezed along its full extent using the thumb and forefinger in a circular motion. The head can be massaged by all the fingers using a circular motion. Whilst the person's head is being supported at the side, the muscles in the neck can be gently massaged, commencing at the top and moving downwards. To exercise the upper chest or pectoral muscles, move the base of the hands from the sternum (breastbone) outwards across these muscles. Both hands can be used to work upwards and also across the stomach area. Once the hands have moved across so that they are under the person's waist, raise the body slightly, thus stretching it.

Another technique for the abdominal area is to glide the hands across but moving in opposite ways. The arm can be massaged by the fingers and thumb and then the fingers can be pressed and gently pulled, with the wrist being held at all times.

Effleurage (as described previously) can be used on the upper leg as far up as the hip on the outside of the leg. Once the person is lying face downwards (with support under the chest), continue to use effleurage movements on the back of the lower leg. Continue as before but work on the upper leg, avoiding the knee. The muscles in the buttocks can be worked upon with both hands to squeeze but making sure that the hands are moving in opposite ways. The foot will benefit from massage using the thumb in small circular movements. For a person suffering from stress or being 'on edge' at the end of a day's work, a back massage can help to ease these problems. With the hands in the position for using effleurage, start the movements at the lowest part of the back and work up and then sideways to the shoulders. The pressure used should be kept up, but as soon as the hands move downwards it should be released. This should be repeated so that all of the back is massaged. Next, using the palms of both hands, work on the top of the shoulder by moving the hands in opposite directions. If the right shoulder is being massaged, the person's head should be turned to the left. The area beside the spine can be massaged, although one should avoid the spinal column. Using both thumbs, one on each side of the spine itself, massage this area by pressing gently in a circle.

Massage has a wide range of uses for a variety of disorders. Its strengths lie in the easing of strain and tension and inducing relaxation and serenity, plus the physical contact of the therapist. Although doctors make use of this therapy in conjunction with orthodox medicine, it is not to be regarded as a cure for diseases in itself and serious problems could occur if this were the case.

Music Therapy

Making music has always been important in all cultures and societies, as a means of self-expression and communication. Many people have experienced the powerful effects of music, which may stimulate feelings of excitement, tranquillity, sadness or joy. Music therapy consists of creating music, using a range of different instruments and the human voice, as a means of helping people to communicate their innermost thoughts, fears and feelings.

Music therapy can help people with a variety of different disorders. It is especially valuable in helping people with intellectual impairment or learning difficulties. However, those who are physically disabled in some way may also benefit, especially people who need to improve their breathing or extend their range of movements.

The sessions are conducted by a trained therapist who has a qualification in music, and the treatment may be available at some hospitals. Many therapists work in residential homes and schools and the demand for the service greatly exceeds the number of people working in this field. The approach taken depends upon the nature of the patient's problems. If the person is a child who is intellectually impaired and who perhaps cannot talk, the therapist builds up a relationship using instruments, vocal sounds and the shared experience of music-making. With a patient who is physically disabled or who has psychological or emotional problems, a different approach with more discussion is likely to be adopted.

Since most people react in some way to music and enjoy the experience of music-making, this form of therapy is usually highly beneficial and successful. Anyone can benefit and the person need not have any previous musical ability, knowledge or experience. Music therapy is especially helpful for children with intellectual and/or physical disabilities.

Naturopathy'

Naturopathy is a holistic approach to healing that centres on an individual person and his or her ability to maintain and restore good health. The techniques used in naturopathy are aimed at helping the body to harness its innate power to heal itself. Naturopaths believe that the body and its functions have a normal, natural balance that maintains good health. Illnesses, which may have a number of different causes, occur when the natural balance is disrupted. Naturopaths are interested in all aspects of a patient and his or her lifestyle rather than concentrating on the symptoms that the person wishes to have cured. The techniques used to bring about healing and maintain good health embrace those of other specialities. They include diet, massage, relaxation and breathing exercises, yoga and meditation, hydrotherapy, osteopathy and chiropractic. The patient is encouraged to take positive steps and be in charge of his or her own health and may need to make changes in lifestyle.

Naturopaths work in private practice and much of the advice and treatment is complimentary to that of conventional medicine. The approach is one of relieving symptoms and promoting good health by adjustments in lifestyle and gentle forms of treatment
when necessary.

Osteopathy

This is a therapy that aims to pinpoint and treat any problems that are of a mechanical nature. The body's frame consists of the skeleton, muscles, joints and ligaments and all movements or activities such as running, swimming, eating, speaking and walking depend upon it. The practice of osteopathy was originated by Or Andrew Still (1828-1917), an American doctor who came to believe that it would be safer to encourage the body to heal itself, rather than use the drugs that were then available and that were not always safe. He regarded the body from an engineer's point of view and the combination of this and his medical experience of anatomy, led him to believe that ailments and disorders could occur when the bones or joints no longer functioned in harmony. He believed that manipulation was the cure for the problem. Although his ideas provoked a great deal of opposition from the American medical profession at first, they slowly came to be accepted. The bulk of scientific research has been done in America with a number of medical schools of osteopathy being established. Or Martin Littlejohn, who was a pupil of Or Still, brought the practice of osteopathy to the UK around 1900, with the first school being founded in 1917 in London.

Problems that prevent the body from working correctly or create pain can be due to an injury or stress. This can result in what is known as a tension headache since the stress experienced causes a contraction in muscles. These are situated at the back of the neck at the base of the skull and relief can be obtained by the use of massage. In osteopathy, it is believed that if the basic framework of the body is undamaged, then all physical activities can be accomplished efficiently and without causing any problems. The majority of an osteopath's patients suffer from disorders of the spine, which result in pain in the lower part of the back and the neck. A great deal of pressure is exerted on the spinal column, and especially on the cartilage between the individual vertebrae. This is a constant pressure due to the effects of gravity that occurs merely by standing. If a person stands incorrectly with stooped shoulders, this will exacerbate any problems or perhaps initiate one. The joints and framework of the body are manipulated and massaged where necessary so that the usual action is regained.

Athletes or dancers can receive injuries to muscles or joints such as the ankle, hip, wrist or elbow and they too can benefit from treatment by osteopathy. Pain in the lower back can be experienced by pregnant women who may stand in a different way due to their increasing weight and, if this is the case, osteopathy can often ease matters considerably. To find a fully qualified osteopath, it is advisable to contact the relevant professional body, or the Doctor. may be able to help.

At the first visit to an osteopath, he or she will need to know the complete history of any problems experienced, how they first occurred and what eases or aggravates matters. A patient's case history and any form of therapy that is currently in use will all be of relevance to the practitioner. A thorough examination will then take place observing how the patient sits, stands or lies down and also the manner in which the body is bent to the side, back or front. As each movement takes place, the osteopath is able to take note of the extent and ability of the joint to function. The practitioner will also feel the muscles, soft tissues and ligaments to detect if there is any tension present. Whilst examining the body, the osteopath will note any problems that are present and, as an aid to diagnosis, use may also be made of checking reflexes, such as the knee-jerk reflex. If a patient has been involved in an accident, X-rays can be checked to determine the extent of any problem. It is possible that a disorder would not benefit from treatment by osteopathy and the patient would be advised accordingly. If this is not the case, treatment can commence with the chosen course of therapy. There is no set number of consultations necessary, as this will depend upon the nature of the problem and also for how long it has been apparent. It is possible that a severe disorder that has arisen suddenly can be alleviated at once. The osteopath is likely to recommend a number of things so that patients can help themselves between treatments. Techniques such as learning to relax, how to stand and sit correctly and additional exercises can be suggested by the osteopath. Patients generally find that each consultation is quite pleasant and they feel much more relaxed and calm afterwards. The length of each session can vary, but it is generally in the region of half an hour. As the osteopath gently manipulates the joint, it will lessen any tenseness present in the muscles and also improve its ability to work correctly and to its maximum extent. It is this manipulation that can cause a clicking noise to be heard. As well as manipulation, other methods such as massage can be used to good effect. Muscles can be freed from tension if the tissue is massaged and this will also stimulate the flow of blood. In some cases, the patient may experience a temporary deterioration once treatment has commenced, and this is more likely to occur if the ailment has existed for quite some time.

People who have to spend a lot of their life driving are susceptible to a number of problems related to the manner in

which they are seated. If their position is incorrect they can suffer from tension headaches, pain in the back and the shoulders and neck can feel stiff. There are a number of ways in which these problems can be remedied such as holding the wheel in the approved manner (at roughly 'ten to two' on the dial of a clock). The arms should not be held out straight and stiff, but should feel relaxed and with the arms bent at the elbow. In order that the driver can maintain a position in which the back and neck feel comfortable, the seat should be moved so that it is tilting backwards a little, although it should not be so far away that the pedals are not easily reached.
The legs should not be held straight out, and if the pedals are the correct distance away the knees should be bent a little and feel quite comfortable.

It is also important to sit erect and not slump in the seat. The driver's rear should be positioned right at the back of the seat and this should be checked each time before using the vehicle. It is also important that there is adequate vision from the mirror so its position should be altered if necessary. If the driver already has a back problem then it is a simple matter to provide support for the lower part of the back. If this is done it should prevent strain on the shoulders and backbone. Whilst driving, the person should make a conscious effort to ensure that the shoulders are not tensed, but held in a relaxed way. Another point to remember is that the chin should not be stuck out but kept in, otherwise the neck muscles will become tensed and painful. Drivers can perform some beneficial exercises while they are waiting in a queue of traffic. To stretch the neck muscles, put the chin right down on to the chest and then relax. This stretching exercise should be done several times. The following exercise can also be done at the same time as driving and will have a positive effect on the flow of blood to the legs and also will improve how a person is seated. It is simply done by contraction and relaxation of the muscles in the stomach. Another exercise involves raising the shoulders upwards and then moving them backwards in a circular motion. The head should also be inclined forward a little. This should also be done several times to gain the maximum effect.

It is possible to give diagnosis and treatment by manipulation, in which the osteopath examines a knee that has been injured. To determine the extent of the problem, the examination will be detailed and previous accidents or any other relevant details will be requested. If the practitioner concludes that osteopathy will be of benefit to the patient, the joint will be manipulated so that it is able to function correctly and the manipulation will also have the effect of relaxing the muscles that have become tensed due to the injury.

Another form of therapy, which is known as cranial osteopathy, can be used for patients suffering from pain in the face or head. This is effected by the osteopath using slight pressure on these areas including the upper part of the neck. If there is any tautness or tenseness present, the position is maintained while the problem improves. It is now common practice for doctors to recommend some patients to use osteopathy and some general practitioners use the therapy themselves after receiving training. Although its benefits are generally accepted for problems of a mechanical nature, doctors believe it is vital that they first decide upon what is wrong before any possible use can be made of osteopathy.

Polarity Therapy

This is a therapy devised by Or Randolph Stone (1890-1983) that amalgamates other healing therapies from both East and West. Or Stone studied many of these therapies, including yoga and acupuncture, and he was also trained to practise osteopathy and chiropractic among others. He began to search for a cure to the problem that he experienced with some of his patients when, although their disorder had been cured by the use of manipulation, they subsequently became unwell. Through his studies of Eastern therapies he accepted the fundamental belief that a form of energy flows along certain channels in the body and that to keep good health the flow must be maintained. In India this energy is referred to as prana and in China it was called chi or qi. The Western equivalent of this would probably be called a person's soul or spirit. It is believed that ailments occur when this flow of energy is blocked or is out of balance, and this could happen for different reasons such as tension or stress, disturbances in the mind or unhealthy eating patterns. This energy is purported to be the controlling factor in a person's whole life and therefore affects the mind and body at all levels. It is believed that once the flow of energy has been restored to normal, the ailment will disappear and not recur.

Dr Stone's polarity therapy states that there are three types of relationships, known as neutral, positive and negative, to be maintained between various areas in the body and five centres of energy.

These centres originate from a very old belief held in India, and each centre is held to have an effect on its related part of the body. The centres are known as ether (controlling the ears and throat), earth (controlling the rectum and bladder),fire (controlling the stomach and bowels), water (controlling the pelvis and glands), and air (controlling the circulation and breathing). The therapy's aim is to maintain a balance and harmony between all these various points, and Dr Stone slowly developed four procedures to do this. They are the use of diet, stretching exercises, touch and manipulation, and mental attitude, that is, contemplation allied with a positive view of life. To cleanse the body from a build-up of toxins caused by unhealthy eating and environmental pollution, the person will eat only fresh vegetables, fruit juices and fresh fruit. The length of time for this diet will vary according to the degree of cleansing required, but it is unlikely to be longer than a fortnight. Also available is a special drink that consists of lemon juice, olive oil, garlic and ginger. After the cleansing is complete, there is another diet to be followed that is said to promote and increase health, and finally one to ensure that the body maintains its level of good health.

Various positions may be adopted for the stretching exercises, such as on the floor with the legs crossed or squatting or sitting with the hands held at the back of the head. It is believed that these exercises free the channels that carry the body's energy and strengthen the sinews, muscles, ligaments and spine. As a way of releasing any stress or tension, the person would be requested to shout out loud at the same time as exercising.

For the first exercise, the person can sit on the floor cross-legged with the right hand taking hold of the left ankle and with the left hand holding the right ankle. The eyes should then be shut and the mind relaxed and quiet.

For the squatting exercise, once in this position, clasp the hands out in front for balance and then move backwards and forwards and also in a circular motion. For people unable to balance in this position, a small book or similar item put under the heels should help.

For a slight change on the basic squatting position, bend the head forward and place the hands at the back of the neck so that the head and arms are between the knees. Relax the arms a little so that they drop forward slightly and thus the backbone is stretched.

Another variation is to hold the hands behind the neck whilst squatting and push the elbows and shoulder blades backwards and inwards. Any tension or stress can be relieved by shouting at the same time as breathing deeply.

Another exercise in which stress can be eased by shouting is known as the 'woodchopper'. This is a fairly simple one to perform, and it entails standing with the feet apart and the knees bent. The hands should be clasped above the head as if about to chop some wood and the arms brought down together in a swinging action ending with the arms as far between the legs as possible. As the hands are being swung downwards, the person should shout, so that any tension is relieved. This action can be repeated quite frequently as long as there is no discomfort.

Touch and manipulation are used by the therapist to detect any stoppages in the flow of energy along the channels, which are believed to be the reason for disorders. It is said that by the use of pressure, of which there are three sorts, the therapist is able to restore the flow of energy. Neutral pressure is gentle and calming and only the tips of the fingers are used.

Positive pressure is the use of manipulation over the whole of the body with the exception of the head. Negative pressure is the use of a firmer and deeper manipulation and touch.

Mental attitude is the fourth procedure, and basically this encourages people to have a more positive view on all aspects of their lives. This is achieved by talking or counselling sessions, and it is believed that a negative view of things can make a person more susceptible to having an ailment. A positive attitude is regarded as being essential for harmony in the body and mind.

Polarity therapy is claimed to be of some benefit to all people who are ill, although it does not concentrate on a particular set of symptoms but is more concerned with the overall aspect of the
patient's health and the achievement of internal harmony and balance. For the therapy to work successfully, each patient has to believe in it completely and be prepared to carry out the practitioner's instructions with regard to diet, exercises, and so on. It is, of course, always advisable to make sure that any therapist is fully qualified before beginning treatment. At the

first consultation, the patient will be required to give a complete case history to the therapist, who will then assess the flow of energy through the body and also check on its physical make-up. Reflexes such as the kneejerk reflex are tested, and any imbalances or blockages in the energy channels are detected by the reflex and pressure point testing. If there is a stoppage or imbalance of the flow, this will be manifested by some physical symptoms. One way in which it is believed a patient can help to speed the restoration of health is by remembering and concentrating on any thoughts, feelings or pictures in the 'mind's eye' that happen while a particular area is being treated. The patient should also have knowledge of the body's ability to heal itself. If a patient is receiving treatment on a painful knee joint, for example, he or she should focus attention on that part of the body whilst being receptive to any feelings that occur.

It is believed that if the patient is aware of the overall condition, as a complete person and not just the physical aspect, this will encourage restoration of health. It is possible that a patient will need to keep details of all food consumed to enable the practitioner to detect any harmful effects, and a 'fruit and vegetable' diet may be advised (as described previously). It may be that the patient has some habit, view or manner of life that is not considered conducive to good health. If this is the case, the patient would be able to take advantage of a counselling service in order to help make a change. Other alternative therapies such as the use of herbal medicine may be used to effect a cure.

Polarity therapy has much in common with other Eastern remedies that have the common themes of contemplation, exercise, touch or pressure, and diet and that can give much improvement. However, it is recommended that an accurate medical analysis of any condition is found in the first instance.

Psychotherapy

Psychotherapy involves exploring and seeking to resolve problems by talking to a professionally trained person who is skilled at helping people to find a way forward through their difficulties. There are many different forms and approaches in psychotherapy, and most involve the person having to delve into his or her inner thoughts and feelings in a process of self-discovery. The psychotherapist guides the person through this process, helping the patient to bring problems to the surface so that they can be examined and resolved. In many cases, there may be deep-seated fears and problems that the patient has suppressed for many years. These may be the cause of the feelings and worries that the person is currently experiencing.

Sessions of treatment in psychotherapy may be on a short or long-term basis depending upon the nature of the patient's problems. Some forms of psychotherapy concentrate on resolving one particular problem with the patient following advice given by the therapist. Usually, these are shorter forms of therapy although it is not unusual for deeper problems to emerge that require further and more lengthy exploration. In all forms of psychotherapy it is important that a good relationship of mutual trust and confidence is built up between patient and therapist. It may be necessary for the patient to consult more than one therapist in the first instance, to find the one with whom he or she feels most at ease.

Modem psychotherapy is largely derived from the work of Sigmund Freud (1856-1939), although there have been many other important workers in this field, developing particular forms of therapy.

Reflexology

Reflexology is a technique of diagnosis and treatment in which certain areas of the body, particularly the feet, are massaged to alleviate pain or other symptoms in the organs of the body. It is thought to have originated about five thousand years ago in China and was also used by the ancient Egyptians. It was introduced to western society by Dr William Fitzgerald, who was an ear, nose and throat consultant in America. He applied ten zones (or energy channels) to the surface of the body, hence the term 'zone therapy', and these zones or channels were considered to be paths along which flowed a person's vital energy, or 'energy force'. The zones ended at the hands and feet. Thus, when pain was experienced in one part of the body, it could be relieved by applying pressure elsewhere in the body, within the same zone. Subsequent practitioners of reflexology have concentrated primarily on the feet although the working of reflexes throughout the body can be employed to beneficial effect.

Reflexology does not use any sort of medication-merely a specific type of massage at the correct locations on the body. The body's energy flow is thought to follow certain routes, connecting every organ and gland with an ending or pressure point on the feet, hands or another part of the body. When the available routes are blocked and a tenderness on the body points to such a closure, then it indicates some ailment or condition in the body that may be elsewhere other than the tender area. The massaging of particular reflex points enables these channels to be cleared, restoring the energy flow and at the same time healing any damage.

The uses of reflexology are numerous, and it is especially effective for the relief of pain (back pain, headaches and toothache), treatment of digestive disorders, stress and tension, colds and 'flu, asthma, arthritis, and more. It is also possible to predict a potential illness and either give preventive therapy or suggest that specialist advice be sought. The massaging action of reflexology creates a soothing effect that enhances blood flow to the overall benefit of the whole body. However, reflexology clearly cannot be used to treat conditions that require surgery.

Reflex massage initiates a soothing effect, to bring muscular and nervous relief. The pressure of a finger applied to a particular point (or nerve ending) may create a sensation elsewhere in the body, indicating the connection or flow between the two points.

This is the basis of reflexology, and although pain may not be alleviated immediately, continued massage over periods of up to one hour will usually have a beneficial effect.

There are certain conditions for which reflexology is inappropriate, including diabetes, some heart disorders, osteoporosis, disorders of the thyroid gland, and phlebitis (inflammation of the veins). *It* may also not be suitable for pregnant women or anyone suffering from arthritis of the feet.

The best way to undergo reflexology is in the hands of a therapist, who will usually massage all reflex areas, concentrating on any tender areas that will correspond to a part of the body that is ailing. However, reflexology can be undertaken at home on minor conditions such as back pain, headache, etc, but care should be taken not to over-massage anyone reflex point as it may result in an unpleasant feeling. Although there have not been any clinical trials to ascertain the efficacy of reflexology, it is generally thought that it does little harm and, indeed, much benefit may result. Some practitioners believe that stimulation of the reflex points leads to the release of endorphins (in a manner similar to acupuncture). These are compounds that occur in the brain and have pain-relieving qualities similar to those of morphine. They are derived from a substance in the pituitary gland and are involved in endocrine control (glands producing hormones, e.g. pancreas, thyroid, ovary and testis).

The body's reflexes

Reflexes on the feet-the soles of the feet contain a large number of zones, or reflexes, that connect with organs, glands or nerves in the body. In addition, there is a 'Small number of reflexes on the top of the foot.

The palms of the hands similarly contain a large number of reflex areas, reflecting to a very large extent the arrangement seen on the soles of the feet. The backs of the hands again mirror, to some extent, the tops of the feet, containing a smaller number of reflex areas.

Use of the hands in reflexology

The hands are considered to have an electrical property such that the right-hand palm is positive and the left-hand palm is negative. The right hand has a reinforcing, stimulating effect while the left has a calming, sedative effect. The back of each hand is opposite to the palm, thus the right is negative and the left is positive. This is important when using reflexology because if the object is to revitalize the body and restore the energy flow that has been limited by a blockage, then the right hand is likely to be more effective. The left hand, with its calming effect, is best used to stop pain.

Reflexes on the body

Reflexes on the body necessarily differ from those on the feet and hands in that there is less alignment with the ten zones. Also, there are a number of reflex points on the body that correspond to several organs or glands. These reflex points are sometimes harder to find accurately and may be more difficult to massage. The middle finger is thought to have the greatest effect so this should be used to work the reflex point. Light pressure should be applied to each point, and if pain is felt it means there is a blockage or congestion somewhere. A painful point should be pressed until the discomfort subsides or for a few seconds at a time, a shorter rest being taken in between the applications of pressure.

The abdominal reflex

A general test can be applied by gently pressing into the navel, either with the middle finger or with one or both hands, with the individual lying in a supine position. The presence of a pulse or beat is taken to mean there is a problem in this area. To combat this, the same technique is used, holding for a few seconds (six or seven), releasing slightly, arid keeping the fingers in the same area, gently massaging with a circular action. If it is necessary to press quite deep to feel the beat, then heavier massage will be required to provide the necessary stimulation.

The same principle can be applied to other reflex points in the abdominal region and the absence of a pulse or beat indicates that there is no problem. In each case, should there be a painful response, holding for a few seconds invokes the sedative action.

Chest reflexes

There are a number of reflex points on the chest relating to major organs in the body. The same massage technique can be adopted for these reflex points as for the abdomen. However, because many of the points lie over bone or muscle, it will not be possible to press in the finger as deeply as for the abdomen. However, pressure should be maintained over tender areas, with a subsequent circular massage, and a similar effect will be achieved.

The techniques and practice of reflexology

Some indication of the massaging, manipulative procedures of reflexology have already been mentioned, but a number of general points of guidance can also be made.

The whole process of reflexology is one of calm, gentle movements in a relaxed state. The foot is probably used most in reflexology in which case shoes and socks and stockings, etc, should be removed. A comfortable position should be adopted on the floor or bed, in a warm, quiet room with the back supported by pillows.

To begin, the whole foot is massaged, indeed both feet should ideally be worked on. However, if working on your own feet it is thought that the right foot should be massaged first (contrary to previous practice). It is considered that the right foot is linked with the past, hence these emotions must be released before the present and future aspects are dealt with in the left foot.

Techniques of massage vary, but a simple method with which to start involves placing the thumb in the middle of the sole of the foot. The thumb then presses with a circular and rocking motion for a few seconds before moving to another reflex. Reference can be made to the diagrams to determine which reflex is being massaged. In all cases, the massage should work beneath the skin, not on the skin. Another method involves starting the massage with the big toe and then moving on to each toe in turn.

In using the thumbs to effect the massage, some refinements of motion can be introduced to give slightly different movements:

I. The thumb can be rocked between the tip and the ball, moving forward over the relevant area. This, along with the circular massage already mentioned, relieves aches and pains.

2. Both thumbs can be used alternately to firmly stroke the skin. This creates a calming effect.

3. The area can be stroked with the thumbs, one moving over the other in a rotational sense. This action is intended to soothe and allow for personal development. In addition to the procedures already mentioned, reflexology can be used to alleviate many symptoms and help numerous conditions. Reflexology can be approached intuitively, so that the pressure of touch and the time factor can vary depending upon response and need.

The use of reflexology

The digestive system

The stomach is an organ that has thick muscular walls and in which food is reduced to an acidic semi-liquid by the action of gastric juice. There are many factors that can cause an upset stomach. To assess the general condition, the stomach body reflex (above the navel) can be pressed. Around it are several related reflexes such as the liver, gall bladder, intestines and colon. The reflex should be pressed for a few seconds and then released three times to activate the reflex.

On *the hands,* the web of soft tissue between the thumb and forefinger of the left hand should be worked with the thumb of the right hand for a few minutes. The hands can be reversed but the stronger effect will be gained this way, because the stomach lies mostly on the left side.

On the feet, the reflexes for the stomach are found primarily on the instep of the left foot although they are also present on the right foot. These should be massaged, but there are further factors, in addition to the use of reflexology, which will aid digestion; these include eating a sensible diet with a minimum of artificial substances, and not overeating. The use of certain essential oils (aromatherapy) can also be of benefit, in this case peppermint oil can often be particularly effective.

The colon is the main part of the large intestine in which water and salts are removed from the food that enters from the small intestine. After extraction of the water, the waste remains are passed on to the rectum, as faeces. If this system becomes unbalanced, then the water may not be absorbed or the food remains pass through the colon so quickly that water cannot be absorbed. In such cases, the result is diarrhoea, which can be painful and inconvenient.

Both body and foot reflexes should be massaged for the stomach, intestines, colon and also the liver and kidneys. The thyroid reflex should also be worked to help regulation of the body functions. A useful body reflex is to press and rotate your finger about two inches above the navel for a couple of minutes. This can be repeated numerous times, each time moving the fingers a little clockwise around the navel, until a complete circuit has been made.

It is important that the condition be stabilized as soon as possible as continued loss leads also to loss of vital salts and a general nutritional deficiency.

At the outset it is possible to work the colon reflexes on the hand to identify any tender areas. The right thumb should be pressed into the edge of the pad (around the base and side of the thumb) of the left palm and worked around to seek out any tender spots. Any tender reflex should be massaged and pressed for a few seconds. In each case, the tenderness should be worked out. Since there are many reflex points crowded onto the navel, it may not solely be the colon reflex that requires some attention. It is always useful to work the reflex on both sides of the body to ensure that a balance is achieved.

A similar approach can be adopted for reflexes on the feet, starting at the centre, or waistline. By applying a rolling pressure, the foot is massaged along to the inner edge and then down the line of the spine and any tender points are worked through pressure and massage. It may be necessary to start with a very light pressure if the area is very tender, and then as the soreness lessens, the pressure can be increased.

Again, diet can be an important factor in maintaining the health of the body and the workings of the colon. Fibre is particularly important in ensuring a healthy digestive system and avoiding ailments such as diverticulitis.

Reflexology can be used for other conditions associated with the digestive system, notably ulcers. A peptic ulcer (in the stomach, duodenum or even the oesophagus) is caused by a break in the mucosal lining. This may be due to the action of acid, bile or enzymes because of unusually high concentrations or a deficiency in the systems that normally protect the mucosa. The result can be a burning sensation, belching and nausea.

To help alleviate the problem, which may be stress-related, the reflexes in the feet should be massaged, as these are often the most relaxing. Obviously the important reflexes are the stomach and duodenum, but it is also worthwhile to work on the liver and the endocrine glands (notably the pituitary). If the ulcer is a longstanding problem or if stomach complaints have been experienced for some time, then further medical help is probably needed.

The heart and circulatory system

The heart is obviously a vital organ. This muscular pump is situated between the lungs and slightly left of the midline. It projects forward and lies beneath the fifth rib. Blood returns from the body via the veins and enters the right atrium (the upper chamber), which contracts, forcing the blood into the right ventricle. From there it goes to the lungs where it gains oxygen and releases carbon dioxide before passing to the left atrium and left ventricle. Oxygenated blood then travels throughout the body via the arteries.

By using body reflexes, the heart can be maintained and conditions can be dealt with by massaging the appropriate reflex points. A useful massage exercise is to work the muscles, rather than the reflex points, of the left arm in a side-to-side movement. This can be followed by the neck muscles and the chest muscles; in each case any tightness or tension should be massaged out. An additional preventative is a good diet, which should be low in fat and cholesterol, but should contain adequate amounts of vitamins, notably the B group, C and E. Exercise is, of course, very important to maintain a good heart and circulation.

There is also a simple test that many reflexologists feel is useful to diagnosing possible heart problems. It may also be worth doing if strenuous activity is contemplated in the near future. Pressure is applied to the pad of the left thumb, at the top. The pressure should be quite hard. It is suggested that when this part of the pad hurts, it indicates a constriction in blood vessels, limiting supply. If the bottom of the pad hurts, this is indicative of congested arteries. If the area is too tender to touch (and there is no physical damage to the hand) then there is a possibility of a heart attack. This test thus provides advance warning and enables a medical doctor to be consulted. Should painful areas occur on both hands, this does *not* indicate a heart problem.

Many blood and circulatory disorders will benefit from the same sort of massage. In these cases the foot reflexes for the endocrine glands (hypothalamus, pituitary, pineal, thyroid and parathyroid, thymus, adrenals, pancreas, ovary or testis) should be worked well, as should those for the circulatory system and heart, lungs and lymphatic system.

Conditions that may benefit from such treatment include:

angina a suffocating, choking pain usually referring to angina pectoris, which is felt in the chest. It occurs when blood supply to the heart muscle is inadequate and is brought on by exercise and relieved by rest. The coronary arteries may be damaged by atheroma (scarring and build-up of fatty deposits). Of particular importance are the heart and circulatory reflexes (veins and arteries) and those of the lymphatic system.

arteriosclerosis a general term including atheroma and atherosclerosis (where arteries degenerate and fat deposits reduce blood flow), which results generally in high blood pressure and can lead to angina. Additional reflexes that should be worked include the liver.

hypertension (high blood pressure) this may be one of several types, the commonest being *essential* (due to kidney or endocrine disease or an unknown cause) and *malignant* (a serious condition that tends to occur in the younger age groups). In addition to the reflexes for the blood and circulation, those for the shoulders, neck and eyes should be worked, in combination with reflexes for the digestive system and liver.

palpitations an irregular heartbeat, often associated with heightened emotions. Also due to heart disease or may be felt during pregnancy. The lung and heart reflexes are particularly important, in addition to those of the circulation. Some heart conditions are very serious and require immediate hospitalization, e.g. cardiac arrest (when the heart stops) and coronary thrombosis. This is when a coronary artery blockage causing severe chest pain, vomiting, nausea and breathing difficulties. The affected heart muscle dies, a condition known as myocardial infarction. However, massage of appropriate reflexes may help, particularly in less serious cases. These should include the heart and circulation (veins and arteries), lungs, endocrine system and the brain. Each will have some beneficial effect in relieving stress and congestion.

varicose veins are veins that have become stretched, twisted and distended, and this often happens to the superficial veins in the legs. The possible causes are numerous and include pregnancy, defective valves, obesity and thrombophlebitis (the inflammation of the wall of a vein with secondary thrombosis). Phlebitis is inflammation of a vein and occurs primarily as a complication of varicose veins. Both these conditions can be treated by massaging the circulatory reflexes and also the leg and liver reflexes (varicose veins themselves should never be massaged). In both cases, resting with the legs in an elevated position is beneficial.

The respiratory system

Asthma is one of the major problems of the respiratory system and its incidence seems to be escalating. The condition is caused by a narrowing of the airways in the lungs. It usually begins in early childhood and may be brought on by exposure to allergens (substances, usually proteins, that cause allergic reactions) exercise or stress.

There are certain body reflexes that can help in this instance. One reflex point is in the lower neck at the base of the V-shape created by the collar bones. Relief may be achieved by pressing the finger into this point with a downward motion for a few seconds. There are additional reflex points on the back, at either side of the spine in the general region of the shoulder blades. These can be worked by someone else with thumb or finger, who should press for a few seconds. Other reflexes that can be worked on the foot include the brain, endocrine glands such as the pineal, pituitary, thymus and thyroid, the lungs, and also the circulatory system.

Particular attention should be paid to the lungs, which includes the bronchi and bronchioles, the branching passageways of the lungs where gaseous exchange (oxygen in, carbon dioxide out) takes place. At the point where the instep meets the hard balls of the feet, and along the base of the lung reflex area is the massage point for the diaphragm. Working the whole of this area will help alleviate symptoms of asthma. During an attack of asthma both thumbs can be placed on the solar plexus reflexes immediately to initiate the soothing process.

The adrenal glands are found one to each kidney, situated on the upper surface of that organ. These are important endocrine glands because they produce hormones such as adrenaline and cortisone. Adrenaline is very important in controlling the rate of respiration and it is used medically in the treatment of bronchial asthma because it relaxes the airways. It is clear therefore, that the adrenal is an important reflex and it is located in the middle of each sole and palm.

Many other respiratory disorders can be helped by using massage of the same reflexes: brain, endocrine glands, lungs and diaphragm, neck and shoulders, augmented by the heart and circulatory system. Conditions responding to this regime include bronchitis, croup, lung disorders and emphysema (distension and thinning, particularly of lung tissue, leading to air-filled spaces that do not contribute to the respiratory process).

Infections of the respiratory tract leading to coughs and colds can also be helped primarily by working the reflexes mentioned above. For colds, the facial reflexes should be massaged, especially that for the nose. However, it is good practice to include the pituitary, and to work the index and middle fingers towards the tip to help alleviate the condition.

With such respiratory problems, there are complementary therapies that can help such as homoeopathy, aromatherapy and Bach flower remedies. There are also many simple actions that can be taken, for example a sore throat may be helped by gargling regularly with a dessertspoon of cider apple vinegar in a glass of water, with just a little being swallowed each time. Honey is also a good substance to take, as are onions and garlic.

The endocrine glands

Endocrine glands are glands that release hormones directly into the bloodstream, or lymphatic system. Some organs such as the pancreas also release secretions via ducts. The major endocrine glands are, in addition to the pancreas, the thyroid, parathyroid, pituitary, pineal, thymus, adrenal and gonads (ovaries and testes).

The endocrine glands are of vital importance in regulating body functions as summarized below: *pituitary* controls growth, gonads, kidneys; known as the master gland *pineal* controls the natural daily rhythms of the body *thyroid* regulates metabolism and growth *parathyroid* controls calcium and phosphorus metabolism *thymus* vital in the immune system. particularly pre-puberty *adrenal* control of heartbeat. respiration and metabolism *gonads* control of reproductive activity *pancreas* control of blood sugar levels

The fact that the endocrine glands are responsible for the very core of body functions means that any imbalance should be corrected immediately to restore the normality. There are some general points relating to massage of these reflex areas. It is good practice to massage the brain reflex first and then the pituitary.

This is because the hypothalamus, situated in the forebrain, controls secretions from the pituitary gland. The pituitary gland then follows. as this is the most important in the endocrine system. The reflexes should be gently massaged with thumb of finger for a few seconds and then gentle pressure exerted and held for a few seconds before releasing slowly.

The pituitary

An imbalance of pituitary gland secretions. often caused by a benign tumour. can lead to acromegaly (excessive growth of skeletal and soft tissue). Gigantism can result if it occurs during adolescence. There may also be consequent deficiencies in adrenal. gonad and thyroid activity. The brain and endocrine reflexes should be worked in order. supplemented by those for the circulation. liver and digestion. In addition to reflex points on the hands and feet. there is also one on the forehead. If any of these reflex areas is found to be tender. it should be massaged often to maintain the balance necessary for healthy growth.

The pineal

The pineal body. or gland. is situated on the upper part of the midbrain. although its function is not fully understood. It would seem. however. to be involved in the daily rhythms of the body and may also play a part in controlling sexual activity. The pineal reflex points are found close to those of the pituitary on the big toes. thumbs and on the forehead and upper lip.

The thyroid

The thyroid is located at the base of the neck and it produces two important hormones. thyroxine and triiodothyronine. Under or overactivity of the thyroid leads to specific conditions.

If the thyroid is overactive and secretes too much thyroxine (hyperthyroidism). the condition called thyrotoxicosis develops. It is also known as Grave's disease and is typified by an enlarged gland. protruding eyes and symptoms of excess metabolism such as tremor. hyperactivity. rapid heart rate. breathlessness. etc. The important reflexes to be worked are the brain and solar plexus. endocrine system and also the circulatory and digestive systems. The reflexes are found on the soles and palms and using the thumbs or fingers. the areas should be massaged. but in stages if the area is very tender.

Under activity of the thyroid. or hypothyroidism. can cause myxoedema producing dry. coarse skin. mental impairment. Muscle pain and other symptoms. In children a similar lack causes cretinism. resulting in dwarfism and mental retardation. The reflexes to be worked are essentially those mentioned for hyperthyroidism. and in addition (for both conditions) the liver reflexes on the right sole and palm should benefit from attention.

There are additional thyroid reflexes elsewhere on the body. notably on the neck roughly midway between jaw and collarbone and on either side. These points should be massaged gently with the thumb and fingers on opposite sides of the throat. Using a gentle gyratory motion. the massage can be taken down to the collarbone. the fingers and thumb of the other hand are then used (on opposite sides of the throat) and the procedure repeated.

Goitre is another condition associated with the thyroid and is a swelling of the neck caused by enlargement of the gland. Typically due to overactivity of the gland to compensate for an iodine deficiency. The important reflexes to concentrate upon are the brain, solar plexus, endocrine system and circulatory system but working of all body reflexes will help.

The parathyroid

There are four small parathyroid glands located behind or within the thyroid. They control the use of calcium and phosphorus (as phosphate) in the body's metabolism. An imbalance of these vital elements can lead to tetany (muscular spasms), or at the other extreme, calcium may be transferred from the bones to the blood, creating a tendency to bone fractures and breaks. The reflexes to these glands are found in the same location as those for the thyroid but it will probably be necessary to massage more strongly to achieve an effect. It is a good idea to work on these areas each time reflexology is undertaken as they are vital in maintaining the metabolic equilibrium of the body.

The thymus

The thymus is located in the neck (over the breastbone) and is a vital contributor to the immune system. It is larger in children and is important in the development of the immune response. After puberty it shrinks although it seems to become more active later in life. Bone marrow cells mature within the thymus and one group, T-lymphocytes, are dependent upon the presence of the thymus. These are important cells as they produce antibodies. The commonest disorder associated with the thymus is myasthenia gravis, which lowers the level of acetylcholine (a neurotransmitter) resulting in a weakening of skeletal muscles and those used for breathing, swallowing, etc. The thymus reflexes are found on the soles of the feet and palms of the hand, next to the lung reflexes. The thymus can also be stimulated by tapping with the finger over its position in the middle of the upper chest.

The adrenals

The two adrenals (also known as suprarenals) are situated one above each kidney and consist of an inner medulla and an outer cortex. The medulla produces adrenaline, which increases the rate
and depth of respiration, raises the heartbeat and improves muscle performance, with a parallel increase in output of sugar from the liver into the blood.

The cortex of the adrenal glands releases hormones including aldosterone, which controls the balance of electrolytes in the body, and cortisone, which, among other functions, is vital in the response to stress, inflammation and fat deposition in the body.

On both the palms and soles, the adrenal reflexes are located above those for the kidneys and if this area is at all tender, it should be massaged for a few seconds. Because the kidney and adrenal reflexes are close together, the massage should be limited to avoid over-stimulation of the kidney reflexes. Disorders of the adrenal glands should be treated by working the endocrine reflexes starting with the pituitary and including the adrenal reflexes, followed by the reflexes for the circulatory, liver and urinary systems.

Specific disorders include Cushing's syndrome, caused by an overproduction of cortisone, which results in obesity, reddening of the face and neck, growth of body and facial hair, high blood pressure, osteoporosis and possibly mental disturbances, and Addison's disease, which results from damage to the cortex and therefore a deficiency in hormone secretion. The latter was commonly caused by tuberculosis but is now due more to disturbances in the immune system. The symptoms are weakness, wasting, low blood pressure and dark pigmentation of the skin. Both these conditions can be treated by hormone replacement therapy but reflexology can assist, through massage of the endocrine, digestive and Liver reflexes.

The gonads

The gonads, or sex glands, comprise the ovaries in women and testes in men. The ovaries produce eggs and also secrete hormones, mainly oestrogen and progesterone. Similarly, the testes produce sperm and the hormone testosterone. Oestrogen controls the female secondary sexual characteristics such as enlargement of the breasts, growth of pubic hair and deposition of body fat. Progesterone is vital in pregnancy as it prepares the uterus for implantation of the egg cell.

The reflexes for these and related organs are found near the ankles on the inside of the feet, just below the angular bone. The same reflex areas are also located on the arms, near the wrist. The ovaries and testes are on the outer edge, while on the opposite, inner edge, are the reflexes for the uterus, penis and prostate. For any disorders that might involve the ovaries or testes, it is also useful to massage other systems such as the brain, other endocrine glands, the circulation and liver.

The pancreas

This is an important gland with both endocrine and exocrine functions. It is located behind the stomach, between the duodenum and spleen. The exocrine function involves secretion of pancreatic juice, via ducts, into the intestine. The endocrine function is vital in balancing blood sugar levels through the secretion of two hormones, insulin and glucagon. Insulin controls the uptake of glucose by body cells and a lack of hormone results in the sugar derived from food being excreted in the urine, the condition known as diabetes mellitus. Glucagon works in the opposite sense to insulin, and increases the supply of blood sugar through the breakdown of glycogen in the liver, to produce glucose.

The primary reflexes for the pancreas are found on the soles and palms, near to the stomach. The thumb should be used, starting on the left foot, working across the reflex area and on to the right foot. If the area is tender, it should be worked until the tenderness goes. Because there are numerous reflexes in this area, there will be stimulation of other organs, to the general wellbeing of the body as a whole.

For other disorders of the pancreas, such as pancreatitis (inflammation of the pancreas) the reflexes associated with digestion should also be worked. Pancreatitis may result from gallstones or alcoholism and, if sufficiently severe, may cause diabetes.

Shiatsu

Shiatsu originated in China at least 2000 years ago, and the earliest accounts gave the causes of ailments and the remedies that could be effected through a change of diet and way of life. The use of massage and acupuncture was also recommended. The Japanese also practised this massage, after it had been introduced into their country, and it was known as *anma*. The therapy that is known today as shiatsu has gradually evolved with time from anma under influences from both the East and West. It is only very recently that it has gained recognition and popularity with people becoming aware of its existence and benefits.

Although East and West have different viewpoints on health and life, these can complement one another. The Eastern belief is of a primary flow of energy throughout the body, which runs along certain channels known as meridians. It is also believed that this energy exists throughout the universe and that all living creatures are dependent upon it as much as on physical nourishment. The 'energy' is known by three similar names, *ki*, *chi* and *prana* in Japan, China and India respectively. (It should be noted that the term energy in this context is not the same as the physical quantity that is measured in joules or calories.) As in acupuncture, there are certain pressure points on the meridians that relate to certain organs, and these points are known as *tsubos*.

Shiatsu can be used to treat a variety of minor problems such as insomnia, headaches, anxiety, back pain, etc. Western medicine may be unable to find a physical cause for a problem, and although some pain relief may be provided, the underlying cause of the problem may not be cured. It is possible that one session of shiatsu will be sufficient to remedy the problem by stimulating the flow of energy along the channels. A regime of exercise (possibly a specific routine) with a change in diet and/or lifestyle may also be recommended. Shiatsu can encourage a general feeling of good health in the whole person, not just in the physical sense. After some study or practice shiatsu can be performed on friends and relatives. There are many benefits for both the giver and the receiver of shiatsu, on a physical and spiritual level.

Energy or ki

There are believed to be a number of auras or energy layers that surround the physical body and that can be detected or appreciated. The first layer, the etheric body, is the most dense and is connected with the body and the way it works. An exercise is described later that enables this layer to be detected. The astral body is much wider, is affected by people's feelings and, if viewed by a clairvoyant, is said to change in colour and shape depending on the feelings experienced. The next aura is the mental body, which is involved with the thought processes and intelligence of a person. Similarly, this can be viewed by a clairvoyant and is said to contain 'pictures' of ideas emanating from the person.

These first three auras comprise the personality of a person. The last aura is known as the causal body, soul or higher self. This is concerned more with perceptive feelings and comprehension. It is believed in reincarnation that the first three auras die with the body but that the causal body carries on in its process of development by adopting another personality. As a person grows in maturity and awareness, these different auras are used, and energy is passed from one layer to another. It therefore follows that any alteration in the physical state will, in turn, affect the other layers, and vice versa.

Seven centres of energy or chakras

It is believed that there are seven main chakras (a chakra being a centre of energy) found midway down the body, from the top of the head to the bottom of the torso. They are situated along the sushumna, or spiritual channel, which runs from the crown of the head to the base of the trunk. Energy enters the channel from both ends. Since the flow is most efficient when the back is straight, this is the ideal posture for meditation or when powers of concentration are required. Each chakra has a component of each aura, and it comprises what is known as a centre of consciousness. Each aura is activated as a person develops, and the same occurs with the chakras, commencing with the lowest (the base chakra) and progressing to the others with time. There is also a change of energy between the auras of each chakra.

The crown chakra is concerned with the pineal gland, which controls the right eye and upper brain and affects spiritual matters. The ajna or brow chakra is linked with the pituitary gland, which controls the left eye, lower brain, nose and nervous system. It has an effect on the intellect, perception, intuition and comprehension. The throat chakra is concerned with the thyroid gland and governs the lymphatic system, hands, arms, shoulders, mouth, vocal cords, lungs and throat. It affects communication, creativity and self-expression. The heart chakra is concerned with the thymus gland and controls the heart, breasts, vagus nerve and circulatory system, and affects self-awareness, love, humanitarian acts and compassion. The solar plexus chakra is concerned with the pancreas. It controls the spleen, gall bladder, liver and digestive system and stomach, and has an effect on desire, personal power and the origin of emotions. The sacral cliakra affects the gonads and controls the lower back, feet, legs and reproductive system. This affects physical, sexual and mental energy, relationships and self-worth.

The base chakra is concerned with the adrenal glands. It controls the skeleton, sympathetic and parasympathetic nervous systems, bladder and kidneys, and affects reproduction and the physical will. As an example of this, if a person is suffering from an ailment of the throat, it is possible that he or she may also be unable to voice private thoughts and feelings.

Zang and fu organs

According to traditional Eastern therapies, organs have a dual function, their physical one and another that is concerned with the use of energy and might be termed an 'energetic function'. The twelve organs mentioned in the traditional therapies are split into two groups, known as zang and fu and each is described below. Zang organs are for energy storage and the fu organs produce energy from sustenance and drink and also control excretion. The organs can be listed in pairs, each zang matched by a fu with a similar function. Although the pancreas is not specifically mentioned, it is usually included with the spleen. The same applies to the 'triple heater' or 'triple burner', which is connected with the solar plexus, lower abdomen and the thorax. The lungs are a zang organ and are concerned with assimilation of energy or ki from the air, which with energy from food ensures the complete body is fed and that mental alertness and a positive attitude are maintained. This is paired with the fu organ of the large intestine, which takes sustenance from the small intestine, absorbs necessary liquids and excretes waste material via the faeces. It is also concerned with self-confidence. The spleen is a zang organ and changes energy or ki from food into energy that is needed by the body. It is concerned with the mental functions of concentration, thinking and analysing. This is paired with the fu organ of the stomach, which prepares food so that nutrients can be extracted and also any energy or ki can be taken. It also provides 'food for thought'. The zang organ of the heart assists blood formation from ki and controls the flow of blood and the blood vessels. It is where the mind is housed and therefore affects awareness, belief, long-term memory and feelings. This is paired with the fu organ of the small intestine, which divides food into necessary and unnecessary parts, the latter passing to the large intestine.

It is also concerned with the making of decisions. The kidneys are a zang organ and they produce basic energy or ki for the other five paired organs and also for reproduction, birth, development and maturity. They also sustain the skeleton and brain and provide willpower and 'get up and go". They are paired with the fu organ of the bladder, which stores waste fluids until they are passed as urine and it also gives strength or courage. The zang organ of the 'heart governor' is concerned with the flow of blood throughout the body. It is a protector and help for the heart and has a bearing on relationships with other people (although there is no organ known as the 'heart governor' it is connected with the heart and its functions). This is paired with the 'triple heater' or 'burner', which passes ki around the body and allows an emotional exchange with others. The liver is the sixth zang organ and it assists with a regular flow of ki to achieve the most favourable physiological effects and emotional calmness. Positive feelings, humour and creativity are also connected with it. The gall bladder is the sixth fu organ with which the liver is paired, and this keeps bile from the liver and passes it to the intestines. It concerns decision-making and forward-thinking.

The Meridian System

The meridians, as previously mentioned, are a system of invisible channels on the back and front of the body along which energy or ki flows. There are twelve principal meridians plus two additional ones, which are called the governing vessel and the conception or directing vessel. Each meridian passes partly through the body and partly along the skin, joining various chakras and organs (the organs as recognized in traditional Eastern medicine). One end of every meridian is beneath the skin while the other is on the surface of the skin on the feet or hands.

Along each meridian are acupressure or acupuncture points, which in shiatsu are called tsubos. These points allow the flow of energy along the meridian to be altered if necessary. The meridians receive energy from the chakras and organs (as described previously), from the meridians with ends located on the feet and hands and also via the pressure points or tsubos. Energy or ki can pass from one meridian into another as there is a 'pathway' linking each meridian to two others. The energy passes in a continuous cycle or flow, and in a set order from one meridian to another. By working on the meridians, and particularly the pressure points, a number of beneficial effects can be achieved with problems such as muscle tension, backache and headache. Since the flow of energy is stimulated by working on the meridians this will, in turn, affect the joints, muscles and skin and thereby ease these complaints. Since a person's mental state, feelings and moods are also altered by the flow of energy, this can induce a more positive frame of mind.

A person in good health should have a constant flow of ki or energy with no concentrations or imbalances in any part of the body. It is believed that the greater the amount of energy there is within a person's body, the greater the vitality, mental alertness and overall awareness that person will possess.

Feeling ki

It is possible for a person to 'feel' ki, and the following exercise helps demonstrate what it is like. Stand upright with the feet apart and the arms stretched upwards. Rub the hands together as if they were very cold, so that a feeling of warmth is generated.

The backs of the hands, wrists and forearms should also be rubbed. The arms should be put down at the side of the body and shaken vigorously. This should then be repeated from the beginning with the arms above the head concluding with the shaking.

Then hold the hands out to the front and they should have a pleasant feeling of warmth and vitality that is due to the circulation of blood and energy that has been generated. The hands should be placed to the sides, then after inhaling deeply concentrate on relaxing as you inhale. This procedure should be done several times and then it should be possible to feel the ki. The hands should be placed about 1m (3.2ft) apart, with the palms of the hands facing inwards. After relaxation, concentrate your thoughts on the gap between your hands and then gradually reduce the space between them; but they must not touch. It is likely that when the hands come quite close, about 15-30cm (6-12ins), a feeling of tingling or warmth may be felt, or the sensation that there is something between the hands. This will be when the auras that surround the hands touch. To reinforce the sensation, the hands should be taken apart again and then closed together so that the feeling is experienced again and becomes more familiar.

The following exercise also enables ki to be felt, but this time the etheric aura around a person's head and shoulders. The previous procedure to generate ki should be repeated, but this time
the hand should be placed near to another person's head, within 60cm-1 m (2-3 .2ft). This person should be sitting upright on the floor or on a chair. The hand should be moved gradually nearer to the seated person's head, concentrating attention on the gap between your hand and their head. If no sensation is felt, the hand should be moved back to its original position, and the process should be repeated.

Again, a feeling of tingling or warmth will probably be experienced as the person's aura is felt. When this has been achieved, the hand can progress round the head and down to the shoulders, noting the edge of the aura at the same time. If the person has no success In experiencing the aura, it is likely that the mind is not clear of other thoughts, so relaxation is suggested prior to any further attempt.

It is also possible for a person, by concentrating their thoughts and by a slight change of position, to alter the now of ki in the body. This will have the effect of either making them feel a lot heavier or lighter, depending on which is desired. Taken to extreme, someone who is ski lieu at the control of ki will prove too heavy to be lifted by four people.

Basic rules

There are some basic rules that should be followed before the practice of shiatsu. Clothing should be comfortable, loose-fitting and made of natural fibres since this will help with the flow of energy or ki. The room should be warm, quiet, have adequate space and be neat and clean. If not, this can have an adverse effect on the flow of ki. The person receiving the therapy should ideally lie on a futon (a quilted Japanese mattress) or similar mat on the floor.

If necessary, pillows or cushions should be ready to hand if the person does not feel comfortable. Shiatsu should not be given or received by someone who has just eaten a large meal; it is advisable to delay for several hours. No pressure should be exerted on varicose veins, or injuries such as cuts or breaks in bones. Although shiatsu can be of benefit to women while pregnant, there are four areas that should be avoided and they are the stomach; any part of the legs from the knees downwards; the fleshy web of skin between the forefinger and thumb, and an area on the shoulders at each side of the neck. Ensure that the person is calm and relaxed. It is generally not advisable to practise shiatsu on people who have serious illnesses such as heart disorders, multiple sclerosis or cancer. An experienced practitioner may be able to help, but a detailed and accurate diagnosis and course of treatment is essential. A verbal check on the person's overall health is important and also to ascertain if a woman is pregnant. If there is any worry or doubt about proceeding, then the safest option is not to go ahead.

Although the general feeling after receiving shiatsu is one of wellbeing and relaxation, there are occasionally unpleasant results such as coughing, generation of mucus or symptoms of a cold; a feeling of tiredness; a headache or other pains and aches; or feeling emotional. The coughing and production of mucus is due to the body being encouraged to rid itself of its surplus foods (such as sugars and fats) in this form. A cold can sometimes develop when the mucus is produced, usually when the cells of the body are not healthy. Tiredness can occur frequently with a person who suffers from nervous tension. After therapy has removed this stress or tension, then the body's need for sleep and rest becomes apparent. A short-lived headache or other pain may also develop for which there are two main reasons. Since shiatsu redresses the balance of ki in the body, this means that blockages in the flow of energy are released and the ki can rush around the body causing a temporary imbalance in one part and resulting in an ache or pain. It is also possible that too much time or pressure may have been applied to a particular area. The amount needed varies considerably from one person to another. However, if a pain or headache is still present after a few days, it is sensible to obtain qualified medical help.

Emotional feelings can occur while the energy is being stimulated to flow, and balance is regained. The feelings may be connected with something from the past that has been suppressed and so, when these emotions resurface, it is best for them to be expressed in a way that is beneficial, such as crying. There may, of course, be no reaction at all. Some people are completely 'out of touch' with their bodies and are only aware that all is not well when pain is felt. If this is so, then any beneficial effects from shiatsu may not register. Due to a modem diet that contains an abundance of animal fats, people become overweight through the deposition of fat below the skin and around the internal organs. The body is unable to 'bum off' this fat and this layer forms a barrier to ki. The flow is stopped and overweight people do not tend to benefit as much due to the difficulty in stimulating the flow of ki in the body.

Exercises and the three main centres

The body is divided into three main centres-the head, the heart and the abdominal centres. The head centre is concerned with activities of a mental nature such as imaginative and intellectual thought processes and is concerned with the brow chakra. The heart centre is concerned with interactions among people and to the world in general including the natural world. It is related to the chakra of the throat and heart. The abdominal centre is related to the base, sacral and solar plexus chakras and is concerned with the practical aspects of life and physical activity. Ideally, energy should be divided equally between the three but, due to a number of factors such as activity, education, diet, culture, etc, this is frequently not so. In shiatsu, more importance is attached to the abdominal centre, known as the *hara.* The following exercise uses abdominal breathing and, by so doing, not only oxygen is inhaled but also ki is taken into the hara where it increases a person's vitality. Once the technique is mastered, it can be practised virtually anywhere and will restore composure and calmness.

Sit on the floor with the back straight and, if possible, in the position known in Japan as *seiza.* The hands should be placed loosely together in the lap and the mind and body should become relaxed after some deep breathing. One hand should be put on the stomach, below the navel, and the other on the chest. When inhaling, this should not be done with the chest but with the abdomen, which should increase in size. As the person exhales the abdomen should contract and this procedure should be practised for a few minutes. After a rest it should be repeated, inhaling quite deeply but still the chest should not be allowed to rise. Some people may not find this exercise at all difficult while others may need more practice. It may be that there is stress or tension in the diaphragm. Once the technique has been mastered, and the hands do not need to be placed on the chest and abdomen, imagine that ki is being inhaled down into the hara. Sit in the same position and inhale slowly via the nose and imagine the ki descending. (It may aid concentration if the eyes are closed.) The breath should be held for about four seconds and concentration should be centred on the ki. Then exhale gradually through the mouth and repeat the process for a few minutes.

The next exercise is known as a centred movement, which practises movement of the ki, since it is one person's ki that should have an effect on another. After practising shiatsu on a partner, you should not feel tired but refreshed and exhilarated. This is a benefit of the extra ki in the body. The exercise should be begun on hands and knees (a body width apart) and it is most important that you are relaxed and comfortable, with no tension. This position is the basis for other movements that are practised on others.

While the position is maintained, begin to move the body backwards and forwards so that you are conscious of the transfer of weight, either on to the hands or knees. The body should then be moved slowly in a circular way, again being aware of the shift of weight from the hands, to hands and knees, to knees, etc, returning to the original position. You should also realize that as the whole body is moved, the abdomen is its 'centre of gravity'.

Practise maintaining a position for about five seconds, registering the increase in weight on the hands when you move forwards and the reduction when you rock backwards. Then return to the original position. It is important that the bodyweight is always used at right angles to the receiver as this will have the maximum effect on the flow of ki. The reason for holding a particular position is that this has the effect of making the person's ki move.

The centred movement previously described can be practised on a partner in exactly the same way, following the same rules. The right hand should be placed on the sacrum, which is between their hips, and the left hand midway between the shoulder blades. As before, you should rock forwards and hold the position for about five seconds and then repeat after rocking backwards on to the knees. This basic procedure can be repeated about twelve times, and if you are not sure whether too much or too little pressure is being used, check with your partner. You will eventually acquire the skill of knowing what amount is right for a particular person.

To summarize, there are some basic rules to be followed when practising shiatsu. A person should make use of bodyweight and not muscular strength and there should be no effort involved. At all times a calm and relaxed state should be maintained and the weight of the body should be at right angles in relation to the receiver's body. The person's whole body should be moved when altering weight on to the receiver, maintaining the hara as the centre. Any weight or pressure held should be for a short time only and both hands should be used equally. It is best to maintain a regular pattern of movement while giving shiatsu and always keep in physical contact with the receiver by keeping a hand on him or her throughout the therapy.

There is a large number of different exercises and techniques, but at each time the giver must be relaxed and calm to enable the flow of ki to occur and thus make the shiatsu work to full effect. As an example, the following exercise on the face and head begins with the receiver's head being held firmly in one hand and, using the thumb of the other hand, press upwards in a straight line between the eyebrows, towards the hairline. Each movement should only be quite small, about 12mm (0.5ins). The fingers should then be placed on each side of the head and the both thumbs used to press from the inner end of the eyebrows towards the hairline. Again, holding the hands at each side of the head, the thumbs should then be used to press from the start of the eyebrows across the brow to the outside.

With the fingers in place at each side of the face, work the thumbs across the bone below the eyes, moving approximately 6mm (0.2ins) at a time. Commencing with the thumbs a little to one side of each nostril, press across the face below the cheekbones. Press one thumb in the space between the top lip and nose and then press with both the thumbs outwards over the upper jaw. Next, press one thumb in the hollow below the lower lip and then press outwards with both puts all fingers of the hands beneath the lower jaw and then leans backwards so that pressure is exerted.

Kyo and Jitsu energy

As a person progresses in the study of shiatsu and comes to understand the needs and requirements of others he or she will gradually be able to give beneficial therapy. It is believed that energy, as previously defined, is the basis for all life, and it is divided into two types known as kyo and jitsu. If the energy is low or deficient it is known as kyo, and if there is an excess or the energy is high, it is known as jitsu. These two factors will therefore affect the type of shiatsu that is given and, with practice, it should be possible to assess visually, and also by touch, what type a person is. A few general guidelines as to how a person can vary his or her shiatsu to suit either kyo or jitsu types are given below. However, as the person progresses, it is likely that an intuitive awareness will develop of what is most suitable for a particular person. For kyo types (low or deficient in energy), a gentle and sensitive touch is required, and any stretched positions can be maintained for a longer time as this will bring more energy to that part of the body. Pressure, held by the thumb or palm, can also be maintained for an increased length of time, approximately 10-15 seconds. For jitsu types (high or excess energy), the stretches can be done quite quickly so that the energy is dispersed, and also shaking or rocking

areas of the body can have the same effect. The pressure that is exerted by the
thumbs or palms should also be held for a shorter length of time, so that excess energy is dispelled.

Yin and yang

As previously mentioned, a change in diet may also be recommended by a shiatsu practitioner. From the viewpoint of traditional Oriental medicine, food can be defined in an 'energetic' way. This differs from the Western definition of foods consisting believed that according to its 'energetic' definition, food will have differing physical, mental, spiritual and emotional effects. This energy is split into two parts, known as yin and yang; yin is where energy is expanding and yang where it is contracting. They are thus opposites and, from traditional beliefs, it was thought that interactions between them formed all manner of occurrences in nature and the whole of the world and beyond. All definitions of yin and yang are based on macrobiotic food (a diet intended to prolong life, comprised of pure vegetable foods such as brown rice), this being the most usual reference. Food can be divided into three main types- those that are 'balanced', some that are yin, and some that are yang. Foods that are defined as being yin are milk, alcohol, honey, sugar, oil, fruit juices, spices, stimulants, most drugs such as aspirin, etc, tropical vegetables and fruits, refined foods and most food additives of a chemical nature. Yang foods are poultry, seafood, eggs, meat, salt, fish, miso, and cheese. Balanced foods are seeds, nuts, vegetables, cereal grains, beans, sea vegetables, and temperate fruits (such as apples and pears).

The balance between yin and yang is very important to the body for example, in the production of hormones such as oestrogen and progesterone, and glycogen and insulin, the expansion and contraction of the lungs, etc. A 'balanced' way of eating, mainly from the grains, beans, seeds, nuts and vegetables, etc, is important as this will help to achieve the energy balance in the meridians, organs and chakras, as defined previously. When these two opposing forces of yin and yang are in harmony and balanced, physical and mental health will result.

Body reading

It is possible for practitioners of shiatsu, as they become increasingly experienced, to assess a person's physical and mental state of health by observing the body and forming accurate observations. If the traditional ways of Eastern diagnosis are studied, this can assist greatly. The Eastern methods were based on the of protein, minerals, fats, carbohydrates, fibre and vitamins. It is senses of hearing, seeing, smelling, and touching, and also by questioning people to obtain information leading to an overall diagnosis. This is known as body reading.

Makko-ho exercises

Makko-ho exercises are six stretching exercises, each of which affects one pair of the meridians by stimulating its flow of energy. If the complete set of exercises is performed, all the body's meridians will have been stimulated in turn, which should result in increased vigour and an absence of tiredness. Before commencing the exercises, you should feel calm and relaxed. It may prove beneficial to perform some abdominal breathing first (as previously described). One example is the triple heater and heart governor meridian stretch. Sit on the ground with either the feet together or crossed. The right hand should grasp the left knee and the left hand the right knee, both quite firmly. Then inhale and, as you exhale, lean forwards and downwards with the top half of the body so that the knees are pushed apart. Hold this position for approximately 30 seconds whilst breathing normally, and then after inhaling return to the upright position. After completion of all exercises, lie flat on the ground for several minutes and relax.

Visualization Therapy

It is now widely accepted that the mind exerts a great deal of influence on the health of the body. People with a cheerful, optimistic outlook on life often experience better health than those who are gloomy and pessimistic. In the case of some serious illnesses such as cancer, it is recognized that people who maintain a positive and determined attitude often do better than those who are passive or fatalistic. In these instances, life in both its extent and quality appear to be affected by the person's state of mind. In visualization therapy it is recognized that the pictures created by the mind (as well as thoughts), can have powerful positive or negative effects on the health of the body. Those using this technique believe that it not only helps people suffering from stress and psychological and emotional problems, but also patients with physical illnesses and symptoms. These include cancer, rheumatic and arthritic disorders and other painful conditions.

In visualization therapy, the patient is first taught the technique of creating a mental image. A person suffering from an emotional or psychological problem is asked to create a picture that is connected with his or her difficulty. The feelings created by the image are explored and discussed with the therapist and changes are made to the picture that, with time, help to resolve the problem. For people with physical illnesses, the image created is often aimed at helping to relieve and ease pain by creating an image of the diseased or painful area and make adjustments to it with the aim' of reducing the impact of the symptoms, though its benefits in the treatment of physical disorders remain controversial.

This form of treatment is normally used with other techniques. It is beneficial for people suffering from stress and emotional problems. Children often respond well to visualization therapy as they are naturally imaginative and find it easy to create mental pictures.

Yoga

From its Indian origins as far back as 4000 years ago, yoga has been continually practised, but it is only in the present century that its use has become more widespread. Yoga has an effect on the whole person, combining the physical, mental and spiritual sides. The word 'yoga' is derived from a Sanskrit word that means 'yoke' or 'union', and thus reflects on the practices of yoga being total in effect. For many hundreds of years in India only a select few, such as philosophers and like-minded people with their disciples, followed the way of life that yoga dictated. The leaders were known as 'yogis' and it was they who taught their followers by passing on their accumulated knowledge. These small groups of people did not live with the people in the villages but dwelt in caves or woods, or sometimes a yogi would live like a hermit. Yoga has had quite far-reaching effects over many hundreds of years in India. The form of traditional healing known as Ayurvedic medicine (see page 37) uses some basic exercises from yoga as part of the treatment.

The basics of yoga were defined by a yogi called Patanjali who lived about 300 BC. He was a very well-respected teacher and commanded great influence at that time, and his classification is one that is used now. He established the fact of yoga being separated into eight different parts. The first two concern a person's lifestyle, which should be serene with the days spent in contemplation, study, maintaining cleanliness, and living very simply and at peace with others. Anything that involve avarice or greed, etc, or is harmful to others has to be avoided. The third and fourth parts are concerned with physical matters and list a number of exercises designed to promote peace and infuse energy into both the mind and body. The remaining four sections are concerned with the advancement of a person's soul or spirit and mental faculties by being able to isolate himself or herself from outside worries and normal life, contemplation and broadening mental faculties with the ultimate knowledge known as somadhi. Mentally, this is a complete change that gives final realization of existence. Much more recently, yoga became available in India to everyone, in complete contrast to centuries ago. Doctors and teachers taught yoga, and it is now the rule that all schoolchildren have lessons in some of the exercises.

Nowadays, the practice of yoga is not restricted to India alone, with millions of people worldwide being followers. There are actually five different types of yoga: raja, jnana, karma and bakti, and hatha. It is this last system that is known in the West, and it involves the use of exercises and positions. The other methods concentrate on matters such as control over the mind, appreciation and intelligence or a morally correct way of life. These other methods are regarded as being of equal importance by the person completely committed to yoga as a way of life. Although people may have little or no spiritual feeling, the basic belief of yoga is the importance of mental attitudes in establishing the physical improvements from exercise. Because of media coverage of a famous violinist receiving successful treatment to a damaged shoulder by yoga, it became very popular throughout the UK. Prior to the 1960s, it was seldom practised, and only then by people who wanted to learn more of Eastern therapies or who had worked and travelled in that area.

It is a belief in yoga that the body's essence of life, or prana, is contained in the breath. Through a change in the way of breathing there can be a beneficial effect on the general health. If a person is in a heightened emotional condition, or similar state, this will have an effect on the breathing. Therefore, if the breathing is controlled or altered this should promote joint feelings of peace and calm, both mentally and emotionally.

There is a variety of exercises, and each promotes different types of breathing, such as the rib cage, shoulder and diaphragm. Some of the movements and stances in use were originally devised from the observation of animals, since they appeared to be adept at relaxation and moved with minimum effort. These stances, which are maintained for one or two minutes, aim to increase freedom of movement and make the person aware of the various parts of the body and any stress that may be present: It is not intended that they be physically tiring or that the person should 'show off' in front of others.

The following twelve stances, known as a greeting to the sun, have the aim of relaxing
and invigorating the body and mind. As suggested by its name. it was originally done when the sun rose and when it set. Although these stances are quite safe. They should not be done by pregnant women or those having a monthly period. except with expert tuition. If a person has hypertension (high blood pressure).

a hernia. clots in the blood or pain in the lower back they are not recommended. Each exercise should follow on smoothly one after the other.

Firstly. stand to attention. hold the palms of the hands together next to the chest with fingers upright. Then inhale and stretch the arms upright with the palms facing the ceiling and lean backwards.

Exhale and. keeping the legs straight. place the fingers or palms on to the ground. Whilst inhaling. bend the knees and place one leg straight out backwards. with the knee touching the ground. In a long, lunging movement. With both hands on the ground, raise the head slightly and push the hips to the front. At the same time as holding the breath, stretch the legs out together backwards, and raise the body off the floor supported by the arms. Exhale and fold the body over bent knees so that the head touches the ground with the arms stretched out in front.

After inhaling and exhaling once, lie face downwards with the body being supported by the hands at shoulder level and also by the toes. The stomach and hips should not be on the ground. After taking a deep breath, stretch the arms and push the body upwards with the head up and the back arched.

Exhale and then raise the hips upwards with the feet and hands being kept on the floor so that the body is in an inverted V-shape. The legs and back should be kept straight.

Exhale and fold the body over bent knees so that the head touches the ground with the arms stretched out in front. Then inhale and move into the position with both hands on the ground, raise the head slightly and push the hips to the front, except that the opposite legs are used from before. Lastly, exhale and place the feet together keeping the legs straight. Bend downwards and place the hands on either side of the feet on the floor, if possible. Inhale and then stand up straight. This whole sequence of exercises forms the greeting or salute and can be performed several times over if wished. If this is the case, it is suggested to alternate the legs used either forwards or backwards in two of the exercises.

It is recommended to follow some simple rules when practising yoga. Firstly use a fully qualified therapist, and practise daily if at all possible. It is advisable to check with a Doctor first if a person is undergoing a course of treatment or is on permanent medication, has some sort of infirmity or feels generally unwell. It is always best that yoga is undertaken before mealtimes but if this is not possible then three hours must elapse after a large meal or an hour after a light one. Comfortable clothes are essential and a folded blanket or thick rug should be placed on the ground as the base. Before commencing yoga have a bath or shower and repeat this afterwards to gain the maximum benefit. It is not advisable to do yoga if either the bowels or bladder are full. If the person is amongst a group under instruction there should be no element of competition. Should the person have been outside on a hot and sunny day it is not recommended that yoga is practised straight afterwards, as feelings of sickness and dizziness may occur.

Yoga is believed to be of benefit to anyone providing that they possess determination and patience. If a person has certain physical limitations then these must be taken into account with regard to their expectation, but there is no age barrier. Teachers believe that people suffering from in stress and disorder in their lives are in greater need of a time of harmony and peace. Yoga was used in the main to encourage health in the physical and mental states and thereby act as a preventive therapy. Tension or stress was one of the main disorders for which it was used, but nowadays it has been used for differing disorders such as hypertension (high blood pressure), bronchitis, back pain, headaches, asthma, heart disorders, premenstrual tension and an acid stomach.

Trials have also been conducted to assess its potential in treating some illnesses such as multiple sclerosis, cerebral palsy, osteoporosis, rheumatoid arthritis and depression experienced after childbirth. Since the effects of tension are often shown by the tightening and contraction of muscles, the stretching exercises performed in yoga are able to release it. Also, being aware of each muscle as it is stretched encourages the person to mentally lose any stress or problems with which they have been beset. Suppleness is developed by the exercises through the use of the bending and twisting actions. This will help to maintain healthy joints, particularly for people who lead rather inactive lives.

The following five stances are ideal for newcomers to yoga, although it may not be possible to do them correctly for some weeks. There should be no strain felt and after practice some or all of them can be done in order. As mentioned previously, it is best to check with a qualified therapist if the person is an expectant mother, suffers from hypertension (high blood pressure), is overweight or is having their monthly period.

The spinal twist entails sitting on the floor with the legs outstretched. The left leg should be bent and placed over the other leg as far as possible. The person should exhale and twist the body to the left. The person's right hand should be moved towards the right foot. The person should have the body supported by placing the left hand on the ground at the back but keeping the back straight. Every time the person exhales the body should be further twisted to the left. The position should be maintained for approximately one minute and then the complete action done again, but this time turning to the right.

The bow entails lying face down on the ground. The knees should be bent and then raised in the direction of the head. The hands should then hold the ankles and, while inhaling, a pull should be exerted on the ankles so that the chest, head and thighs are raised up away from the floor. To start with it will not be possible to hold the legs together, but this will gradually occur with regular practice. This position should be maintained for up to ten breaths. To complete the bow, exhale and let go of the legs.

The half shoulder stand involves lying on the back with the legs raised during inhalation. At the same time as exhaling, the hips should be lifted and the legs moved so that they pass over the head. The body's weight should be taken by the shoulders, elbows and arms. Upon inhaling, the legs are moved so that the hands do not feel uncomfortable with the weight. This stance should be maintained for a few minutes (perhaps one minute at the start) while breathing in a normal manner. The arms should be returned to the floor and the person should inhale whilst letting the body gradually return to the floor in a rolling action.

The bridge this stance is carried out on the floor, starting with the person lying on the back, the knees should be bent, with the legs separated a little and the arms at the side of the body. The person should then inhale and lift the torso and legs, thus forming a bridge. The fingers should then be linked under the body and the arms held straight. The person should then incline the body to each side in turn, ensuring that the shoulders stay underneath. To make the bridge a little bigger, pressure can be exerted by the arms and feet. After inhaling, the position should be maintained for a minimum of one minute and the body returned to a relaxed normal position on the floor.

The triangle commences with the person standing upright with the legs apart and the arms held out at shoulder level. Extend the right foot to the side and, upon exhaling, bend over the right-hand side so that the right hand slips downwards in the direction of the ankle. There should be no forward inclination of the body at this time. As the bending action takes place, the left arm should be lifted upright with the palm of the hand to the front. This stretched position should be kept up for the minimum of a minute, with the person trying to extend the stretch as they exhale. After inhaling, the person should then revert to the beginning of the exercise and do it again but leaning in the opposite direction.

As previously mentioned, yoga has recently been used to treat some illnesses such as rheumatoid arthritis, and if a person has such a severe disorder, then a highly skilled and experienced therapist is essential. Since this form of yoga, known as therapeutic yoga, is so new there is only a limited number of suitably experienced therapists available, although this situation should be remedied by the introduction of further training. For those who wish to use yoga to maintain mental and physical health, joining a class with an instructor is perhaps the best way to proceed, so that exercises are performed correctly and any lapses in concentration can be corrected. These classes last usually in the region of an hour and are separated into sessions for beginners and those who are more proficient. Proficiency and progress is achieved by frequent practice, which can be done at home between lessons. One simple exercise that helps reduce stress is quite simple to perform and does not take long. The person should lie on the floor with the arms at the side and the legs together. After inhaling, all the muscles from the toes to the thighs should be tightened in turn. As the person exhales, the muscles in the stomach up to the shoulders should then be tightened, including the hands, which should be clenched. After inhaling again, the chest, throat and face muscles should be tightened, as well as screwing up the face and this should be maintained until the next breath has to be taken. All muscles should then be relaxed, the legs parted and the arms spread out comfortably with the palms facing the ceiling. The person should then totally relax with a sensation of falling through the ground.

The majority of doctors regard yoga as a type of exercise that is beneficial, although some do recommend patients to refer to yoga practitioners. However, if a specific disorder is to be treated, it is very important that the ailment should first be seen by a doctor.

www.ingramcontent.com/pod-product-compliance
Lightning Source LLC
Chambersburg PA
CBHW070747310526
45791CB00029B/1788

* 9 7 8 1 5 1 5 0 1 5 3 2 1 *

worldwide, facilitate information exchange, and support social, personal, and business interactions.

b) **Information Access**: Electronics provide access to an abundance of information. This empowers individuals with knowledge and educational resources, facilitates research, and supports lifelong learning.

c) **Healthcare**: Electronics are vital in modern healthcare. They enable advanced medical equipment, telemedicine, electronic health records (EHRs), and remote monitoring, improving patient care, diagnosis, and treatment.

d) **Entertainment**: Electronics drive the entertainment industry, from high-definition TVs and gaming consoles to streaming services, music players, and virtual reality. They offer a wide range of options for leisure and relaxation.

e) **Transportation**: Electronics enhance transportation with innovations like GPS navigation, advanced driver-assistance systems (ADAS), and electric vehicles. They improve safety, reduce environmental impact, and increase efficiency.

f) **Energy Efficiency**: Electronics contribute to energy efficiency through smart grids, energy-efficient appliances, and renewable energy technologies. They help reduce energy consumption and lower environmental impacts.